LIVING BUDDHISM

LIVING BUDDHISM

Mind, Self, and Emotion in a
Thai Community

JULIA CASSANITI

CORNELL UNIVERSITY PRESS
ITHACA AND LONDON

First published 2015 by Cornell University Press
First printing, Cornell Paperbacks, 2015

Printed in the United States of America

Library of Congress Cataloging-in-Publication Data

Cassaniti, Julia, author.
    Living Buddhism : mind, self, and emotion in a Thai community / Julia Cassaniti.
        pages cm
    Includes bibliographical references and index.
    ISBN 978-0-8014-5400-4 (cloth : alk. paper) —
    ISBN 978-0-8014-5671-8 (pbk. : alk. paper)
    1. Health—Religious aspects—Buddhism. 2. Buddhism—Thailand—Chiang Mai. 3. Chiang Mai (Thailand : Province)—Social life and customs. I. Title.
    BQ4570.M4C37   2015
    294.3′9109593—dc23   2015014598

Cloth printing   10 9 8 7 6 5 4 3 2 1
Paperback printing   10 9 8 7 6 5 4 3 2 1

To Elsie and Joseph Perrone

CONTENTS

Part III. Karma

ACKNOWLEDGMENTS

This book has benefited from the support of so many people; I would like to thank them here. My advisers at the University of Chicago, Richard Shweder, Steven Collins, Tanya Luhrmann, and Richard Taub, have helped me to think and grow the ideas in this book through countless conversations and have been a great source of sustained intellectual encouragement through the years. Richard Shweder has helped me to think deeply about psychological diversity and the worth of leaving no assumption unquestioned in revealing the social construction of what counts as normal. In discussions ranging from the Buddha's hurt toe to the politics of female monk ordination, Steven Collins has helped me think about Buddhism as a living, moving mix of practices, as true when the Buddha was teaching as it is now. Tanya Luhrmann has helped me think carefully about the relationship between attention and thought in religious (and psychological) practice, and has reminded me how far good writing can go in sharing ideas and insights. Richard Taub, through institutional and personal backing, has helped me remember how much the support of mentors is crucial to success. In addition to these advisers I would like to also and especially thank George Robinson, who as my undergraduate adviser at Smith College believed in me and fostered the intellectual curiosity that made this book possible.

Friends in Chiang Mai enabled my writing of this book by housing me literally and intellectually during my years of passing through the city. These friends include Piyawit Moonkham, who first brought me to Mae Jaeng; Uthen Mahamid, who reminds me to think outside the box; Gaewgarn Fuangtong, my constant go-to English speaker and Bangkok-Chicago contact; Thongsuk Mongkhon, who shares his home with me when I'm in town; Pussadee Nonthacumjane, who makes her library and classes at Chiang Mai University available for my use; and Aj. Somwang Kaewsufong, who is always available to help me with Thai Buddhist studies questions. They have all contributed to this work through their constant support, aiding in everything from figuring out the best motorbike helmet to buy, to digging up local histories of Northern Thai spirit cults.

I would also like to thank members of the various institutions I have been affiliated with and the granting agencies that have lent their support during the writing of this book. They include Katherine March at Cornell University, who introduced me to anthropological research years ago and has continued to be a great personal and professional mentor; Thak Chaloemtiarana and members of the Kahin Center Southeast Asian Studies Program, who provided a wonderful place to write; Thomas Csordas, Janis Jenkins, and the Anthropology Culture and Medicine Seminar at the University of California, who inspired me to think harder about cultural meanings and their connections to health; Tanya Luhrmann at Stanford University, who served as my Culture and Mind postdoc adviser; and Jocelyn Marrow, Jeanne Tsai, Hazel Markus, and the Psychology Department's Culture Co-Lab, who together pushed me to think further about the psychological implications of my research; the Cultural Anthropology with a Hint of Psychological Anthropology Reading Writing Group at Washington State University has similarly helped to improve the ideas and the writing in its final stages. The National Research Council of Thailand, the Fulbright Foundation, the Mellon Foundation, the Department of Comparative Human Development, the Committee on Southern Asian Studies, and the Institutional Review Board at the University of Chicago have all provided financial and institutional confidence at times when either or both were getting low. Peter Potter, Max Richman, Ange Romeo-Hall, and the whole editorial team at Cornell University Press have been a pleasure to work with from start to finish.

My parents Jackie and Joseph Cassaniti, my brother Jarret, and my sister Jocelyn have all been so incredibly supportive of the time and research that went into this book, reading drafts and offering suggestions throughout the long process of development to finished product. I really can't thank them enough. I would also like to thank friends and colleagues who have read sections or full manuscript drafts and have otherwise offered material and immaterial support for the work over the years: Jessica Auerbach, Jason Chung, Laura Darlington, Andrew Dicks, Rachel Dunn, Barb Dybwad, Nancy Eberhardt, Eli Elinoff, Rebecca Hall, Jacob Hickman, Jeff Holt, Jeannette Mageo, Tian-Tian Mayimin, Jessica McCauley, Justin McDaniel, Matthew Newsom, Brooke Schedneck, and Benjamin Smith. Bianca Dahl, Justin Van Elsberg, Scott Stonington, Emily Zeamer, and two anonymous reviewers have read through and helped to improve full manuscript drafts. Each of these friends has offered invaluable suggestions to the work as it has taken shape. I'm extremely grateful to all of them.

Finally, I would like to thank especially the people of Mae Jaeng who are the subject of this book. It would not be here without the help of these friends, especially those I call Sen, Goy, Duansri, and their friends and families, along with my research assistant Ari Chuchuhnjitsakul. I have changed the names of those in Mae Jaeng to protect their privacy, and in doing so I can't adequately thank them here, but their kindness in opening up their lives to me has been an indelible part of my own journey.

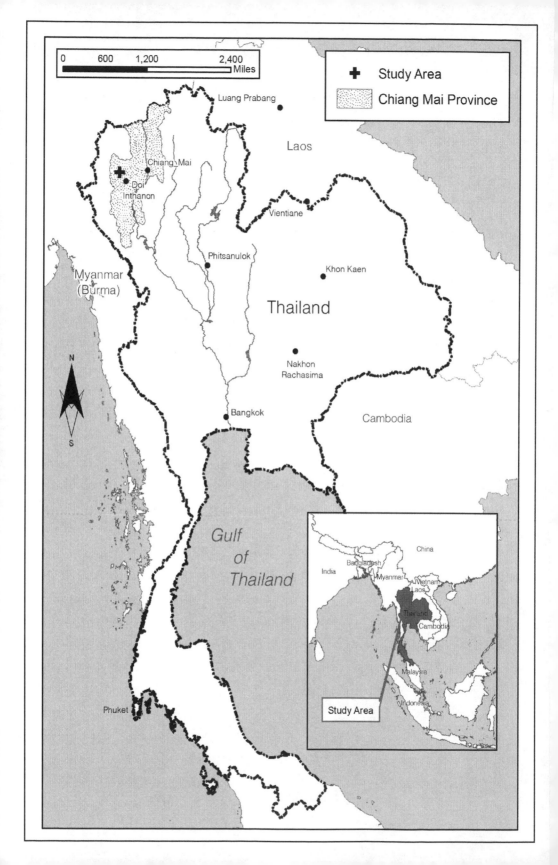

Central Characters

Goy's family

Goy: A thirty-three-year-old woman who owns a stationery store in Mae Jaeng[1]

Mae Daeng: Goy's fifty-six-year-old mother and my host mother, owner of a market stall

Ta: Goy's twenty-four-year-old brother, unemployed

Gaew's family and friends

Gaew: A thirty-year-old woman, whose family runs a general goods store in Mae Jaeng

---

1. Selected place names and names of people described are pseudonyms. Some slight additional characteristics have been changed to ensure privacy, but the general area of Northern Thailand, the quotes, and relevant facts about the place and people are all true to life. Ages stated reflect ages at the beginning of extended fieldwork in 2005–6, three years after the author's first visit to Mae Jaeng in 2002 and two years before Sen's hospitalization in 2007.

Sen: Gaew's thirty-two-year-old brother, and the subject of the book's extended case study

Noi: Sen and Gaew's eleven-year-old brother

Mae San: Their fifty-one-year-old mother

Paw Nui: Their fifty-five-year-old father

Pan: Gaew's thirty-one-year-old husband

Chai: A twenty-nine-year-old man, owner of a medical clinic, and Sen's close friend

Aung: A thirty-year-old woman, a pork vender at the market, and a friend of Gaew and Sen

Duansri: A thirty-two-year-old woman living in the nearby Karen Christian village of Ban Ko Tao

Julia: Thirty-one-year-old woman, anthropologist, and narrator of this book

KEY TERMS

anicca: Impermanence (Pali; in Thai, *anitchang*), one of the Three Characteristics of life in Buddhist thought, along with *dukkha* (*dukkhang*, nonsatisfactoriness) and *anatta* (nonself)

dhamma: (Pali; in Thai, *dham*; in Sanskrit, *dharma*) the Buddhist teachings

jai: (Thai) heart-mind, the seat of emotion used in compound words, including *jai yen* (cool-hearted, calm), *jai ron* (hot-hearted, impatient), and *kreng jai* (deferential, awe-struck)

kamma: Karma (Sanskrit)/*kamma* (Pali), the Buddhist theory of a natural moral cause and effect based on intention

tham jai: (Thai) to make the heart, acceptance

wat: A Thai Buddhist monastery

See glossary for more terms.

Living Buddhism

PROLOGUE

Mae San and Paw Nui stared at the wall absently, not seeming to know where to focus. They hadn't slept in three days, other than some short naps on the hard seat of the Chiang Mai hospital waiting room. Their daughter Gaew paced back and forth in the room, sitting down and then standing up again to go over to the hospital bed to check on her brother, Sen, who lay half awake. Every few minutes Sen would sit up, the tubes that were connected to him moving with him as he did. He reached out with his index finger and thumb to flick away the ash of an imaginary cigarette. Gaew adjusted the tubes and continued pacing. After a while the doctor finally came in, and Mae San and Paw Nui stood up to greet him.

"His liver is shot," the doctor said. "I'm sorry, there's nothing more we can do. We could try keeping him here and see if he improves, but I doubt it." Mae San and Paw Nui sat back down. A little while later a nurse came over. "I've seen this before," she told us. "You have to *tham jai*, you have to make your heart. Bring him home, let him be comfortable." Mae San, Paw Nui, and Gaew discussed the matter, and soon Sen was loaded back into the ambulance that had brought him into the city, and returned to Mae Jaeng over the mountains outside Chiang Mai. Once Sen was back at the Mae Jaeng hospital, his friends gathered around his bed, Sen lying almost completely unconscious, his wrists and legs tied so he couldn't move. The town's ghost doctor, Nan Jon, came in to detach the spirits of alcohol from his body, and the town's main medical doctor, Moh Bom, gave him medicine.

"*Tong ploy*," his family and friends told each other that night; "We have to let go." They said it half in a daze as they ate grilled pork and birthday cake at Mae Jaeng's only restaurant. It was Sen's thirty-fifth birthday, and his brother Noi's twelfth birthday too, but no one was in a mood to celebrate. "It was his karma," they said to each other, to me, to themselves. "People are born, they grow, they hurt, and they die." They went to their local Buddhist monastery to make merit. Later, back at the hospital, I talked to Moh Bom. "We should have done something sooner!" I said, distraught. "Julia . . ." he replied, "*anicca*. Do you know *anicca*? It means that everything is impermanent. You have to make your heart."

I didn't understand what he meant. I didn't feel like I understood any of it. The expectations that the people around me had about Sen and about health in general seemed to clash with my own cultural ideas formed while growing up in a liberal upstate New York town. I wanted to think about what had happened, and to figure out what could have been done differently. I wanted to understand the anguish that I and (what it seemed to me) everyone else were feeling. In the hospital the only friend of Sen other than me who seemed upset at all was Daeng, who had just flown in from England, where she had been living with her British husband.

"Why didn't they make him stop drinking earlier?" she asked me, crying. I felt the same way, but it seemed to me that we were the exceptions. In contrast, Sen's friends and family were saying that we should all calmly accept what was happening. They talked about impermanence, and karma, and a lot about making the heart.

"Making the Heart" (*tham jai*) is a popular idiom heard regularly in Thai and often translated into English as "acceptance." It is not a phrase often related in scholarship to Buddhist philosophy. Through interviews, observations of religious ritual, and close participation in everyday life, however, I came to realize that practices of "making the heart" deal centrally with Buddhist ideas about the importance of being aware of change (in the sense of the Pali word *anicca*, or impermanence) and the "letting go" of affective attachments.

This book is about making the heart in Mae Jaeng. I show how ideas about the heart are understood, interrelated, and reinforced through secular and religious practices in the course of everyday life. I start by recounting the state of emotional and religious life in the community; I then develop a narrative that untangles the feelings, problems, and solutions of Sen and his family and friends in the year leading up to his hospitalization in 2007. In the process, I reveal a psychological orientation to health and well-being in the community that looks quite different from what one might find in many of the scholarly accounts in the psychological sciences, Buddhist studies, and anthropology of religion.

I had studied psychology as an undergraduate at Smith College, and while traveling and working in a dozen countries in Asia I started wondering whether the psychological tenets I had studied in college were more or less universal than I had been taught. I wondered if they weren't more a part of a cultural psychology that spoke to particular times and places in the United States, but that did not adequately address the world's psychological diversity. I was reading about Buddhism as I traveled in Asia, and the more I read and experienced Buddhist ideas, the more it seemed that there was something significant about the way the world is understood according to Buddhist teachings, teachings that everywhere seemed to profess universality but that demonstrated variation more dependent on *where* the Buddhist practices occurred. After my travels I enrolled in the Comparative Human Development program at the University of Chicago for my PhD to learn more about the cultural psychology of Buddhism in practice.

I knew the country where I wanted to do my research, but I didn't know a place to base myself. Then I heard about a fairly typical, remote valley community called Mae Jaeng, where the villagers were still very much rooted in tradition. People told me in hallowed tones that life there was pure and "really Thai"—far removed from the modern but degenerate experience of urban living. "But you know, people out in the countryside like in Mae Jaeng," one Chiang Mai man told me, leaning back in his chair having overheard me at a coffee shop talking about the possibility of going there, "they don't really understand Buddhism, it's too difficult and abstract for them." He paused, and seeming to change his mind, he continued: "But even though they don't know it, they really *get* it. They don't know how to say it, but they *understand* it, they live it. They're in touch with the earth, they don't know, but they *know* . . . more than city people." The man seemed to be lost in some image of a nostalgic golden past, imagining a time and place where people were ignorant but wise, understanding things they couldn't articulate. After spending months around the hip coffee shops of Chiang Mai, I was curious. What would people think, and how would they live, in such a so-called "backward" but "pure" place?

A Thai man named Piyawit had been to Mae Jaeng, and as he was between jobs and eager to learn English, he agreed to take me there. We were warned in Chiang Mai: "It's the rainy season. Be careful driving. You shouldn't go." But we headed out on my motorbike anyway, up over the mountains two hours from Chiang Mai city and down the slippery other side, into a lush valley that seemed to grow around us in the mist. Piyawit helped me find the only hotel in town, a kind of byway for truckers staying over on the supply road from Mae Hong Son in the far north to Chiang Mai city. Within a few days he had helped me find a balcony attached to a house by some rice fields in a back village to rent for two months. After introducing me to a man who knew a little bit of English to help me with interviews, he returned to Chiang Mai.

The research that began that summer continued through multiple extended visits to Mae Jaeng over the course of ten years, two months out of every year beginning with that visit in 2002 and concluding in 2012, with eighteen months of continuous fieldwork between May 2005 and December 2006. I carried out ethnographic data collection, especially making use of its participant observation methodology, in order to develop understandings about Buddhism in practice. Participant observation has allowed me to get past assessments of psychological life of the kind usually conducted in laboratory experiments and through large-scale surveys on college campuses, the kinds of studies that strive to isolate variables from their real lived experience. I chose to live in a community, get to know the people in it, and learn from them as they lived their lives. To that end I have slept in the homes of people in Mae Jaeng, eaten their food, taken trips with them, and accompanied them as they harvested rice and gathered water and replenished their shops. I experienced their ordinations, graduations, relationships, and their personal, social, and economic activities. Between field trips I maintained connections with friends and contacts in Mae Jaeng through Facebook, phone, and video calls. Gaew, Sen, Goy, and the others I came to know in Mae Jaeng have become some of my closest friends. This book is about what I learned of Buddhist practice and the cultural psychology of making the heart in Mae Jaeng during the ten years I have gotten to know them.

INTRODUCTION

A World of Change

I first met Goy in my daily walks past her shop as I crossed from the farming village of Ban Hai on the edge of town to the town center in Mae Jaeng, where I was interviewing people about Buddhism. Often I would stop outside Goy's dusty stationery store and sit down on the mats she had laid outside, and get a drink of water or have a snack, resting after walking through the fields from Ban Hai, before crossing the bridge of the Mae Jaeng River and heading into the market. Back then I couldn't speak Thai very well, and Goy's English was almost nonexistent, but we managed to talk and relax together almost daily in my first months in town. Goy was about my age, a graduate of the accounting department at a nearby university. She didn't smile much, but when she did it was genuine and kind, and she liked to talk about Buddhism.

One afternoon she told me about her father: "He was a police chief here in Mae Jaeng," she said, "and then he died. Almost a year ago."[1] He was

---

1. All quotes are translations from Thai unless otherwise noted. I follow a modified version of the Royal Thai General System in most cases, unless otherwise preferred by popular precedent

forty-seven and apparently healthy. She explained that he had been sitting outside with the family at a fire, having dinner, when suddenly he stopped breathing. A heart attack had killed him almost instantly. Goy and her family were still recovering from the shock when I met her.

In our conversations Goy told me about how she had dealt with the loss, and how hard it had been on her and her family. "I mean, he was there, and then he wasn't," she told me, looking at me as if it was a lesson of some kind. "It was really hard on my little brother and my mother and me. At that time I was interested in Buddhism, but after he died I started reading more about it, more *dhamma* books [teachings of the Buddha]." "Especially," she continued, "I started learning more and more about the idea of *anicca*, of impermanence. Now we can laugh, speak, and breathe, but how about tomorrow? Can we do this tomorrow? No one can answer. This leads one to doing everything carefully. We don't know if there will be time for us later."

I had learned the Pali word *anicca* (pronounced, roughly: ahn-IHT-cha) from my own study of Buddhism, but I didn't know much about it. Goy showed me a book that explained more. *Anicca* refers to instability, or change. "It means that nothing stays the same," Goy said, pointing to a *dhamma* book that describes it as one of the "Three Characteristics" (or in the Pali language of Theravada Buddhism the *tilakkhana*) of existence, along with *dukkha* (suffering, or non-satisfactoriness) and *anatta* (the idea that there is no such thing as a stable self).[2] "When I started to think of *anicca*," Goy said, "I started to feel better about what happened to my dad."

(e.g., *jai* instead of *chai*, and *mae chee* instead of *mae chii*) or by my informants' preferences (for personal and place names). Italicized quotes represent word-for-word translations based on audio recordings; other quotes are reconstructed from notes taken at the time or in field notes the day they were spoken. In many of the translated passages I have repeated a Thai or Pali term or phrase in English, or vice versa, in order to avoid overuse of bracketed interpolations.

2. Pali is the formal religious language of Theravada Buddhism; it is a religious lingua franca comparable to the role of Latin in English. There is no unique script for Pali; instead it is written in local scripts, with Roman characters by English speakers and in Thai characters by Thai speakers. Hundreds of Pali words have infiltrated the everyday vernacular of the Thai language, with slight variations on pronunciation: the English word "karma," for example, is a Sanskrit word that is called *kamma* in Pali and *kam* in Thai, and the word for dharma is *dhamma* in Pali and *dham* in Thai. In the United States, Sanskrit-based words are more commonly known: karma (in Pali, *kamma*) and dharma (in Pali, *dhamma*) are two examples. Although it is thought that the Buddha himself spoke neither Sanskrit nor Pali, teaching instead in a related local language of his region, Sanskrit has come to be associated with the northern "Mahayana" Buddhist schools of China, Tibet, Korea, and Japan and is more well-known in the United States, while the older Pali language is found in the southern "Theravada" schools of Thailand, Sri Lanka, Burma, Cambodia, and Laos.

Anicca is an idea with a long and complex history. It is part of a long tradition of Buddhist thought, and like Buddhism in general it is practiced in Mae Jaeng as part of a complex web of everyday life in the community. *Anicca* most closely relates to its place as one of the Three Characteristics of human, non-enlightened life, along with *dukkha* and *anatta*. More broadly it refers to ideas that underscore the whole of Buddhist teaching. The Buddha is thought to have taught his *dhamma* (Sanskrit, *dharma*) somewhere in what is today northeastern India about twenty-five hundred years ago, after becoming disillusioned by the inevitable human condition of sickness, old age, and death. Today it is estimated that 7 percent of the world's population, and 95 percent of the people in Thailand, follow the Buddha's teachings.[3] In reaching enlightenment (*nibbana*; Sanskrit, *nirvana*), the Buddha taught that life is suffering, and that the cause of suffering is craving. He taught that life is characterized by attachments and wishes for things that will necessarily bring suffering because of their impermanent nature. These wishes especially include the wish for a permanent self, even as a stable self cannot be found. He taught that the underlying intentions of one's action accumulate as a moral force called *kamma* (usually known in English by its Sanskrit form, *karma*) that follows one through multiple lives. Through what has come to be referred to as these "Noble Truths," the Buddha laid out a practical and philosophical plan for the development of morality, concentration, and wisdom.[4]

In many respects Buddhism in Thailand looks like Buddhism everywhere in emphasizing these ancient ideas, whether they take the form in practice of northern traditions like Zen or Tibetan, or of other Theravada traditions like those found in Sri Lanka, Burma (Myanmar), Cambodia,

---

3. Global statistics are from the Pew Research Center's forum on Religion and Public Life—Global Religious Landscape 2012, at http://www.pewforum.org/2012/12/18/global-religious-landscape-exec/. Thai statistics are from the 2000 Thai census, at http://www.religionfacts.com/religion_statistics/religion_statistics_by_country.htm.
4. This plan is known as the "Eightfold Path" and is part of the "Four Noble Truths" that make the foundation of Buddhist thought. The Four Noble Truths are (1) the fact of non-satisfactoriness (Pali *dukkha*, often also translated as suffering, anxiety, stress, or dissatisfaction); (2) the cause of non-satisfactoriness (the cause of *dukkha* is *tanha*, craving); (3) the cessation of non-satisfactoriness (this is also known as *nibbana*, or nirvana, the goal of Buddhism); and (4) the path leading to the cessation of non-satisfactoriness (known as the Eightfold Path, involving wisdom, ethical conduct, and concentration). See Rahula 1974 for further explanation on this and Buddhist teachings in general.

and Laos, or through the many diasporic and non-Asian Buddhist communities springing up through the global transmission of people and
ideas.[5] Regardless of place, those who follow Buddhism may choose to
become a renunciate monk, joining the Buddhist Sangha (the official
monastic order)[6] as a *bhikkhu* (a male monastic), or, less commonly, a *bhikkhuni* (a female monastic). Or they may participate in religious rituals as
a lay follower by making offerings or paying homage to the teaching. Or
they may just agree with and aspire to emulate the Buddha's lessons, which
for many includes following a set of guidelines for living called the Five
Precepts, which entail abstaining from killing, stealing, lying, intoxication,
and sexual misconduct, with a good deal of variation in practice according
to personal and social interpretations. While the official Sangha at the local
and national levels monitors the activity of the ordained, and defrocks those
found to be in violation of the much more numerous precepts required for
monastics, for lay followers there is no body of authority to declare someone a "good" or "proper" or even "real" Buddhist. Buddhism is very much
considered a moral practice, and people regularly interpret and comment
on their own and others' behaviors, but overall people are considered Buddhist if they declare themselves to be, regardless of their interpretations
and expressions of Buddhist teachings.

Buddhist practice in Thailand looks similar in many respects to Buddhism everywhere, but it takes on its own unique forms through engagements with long and complex religious, political, and social histories. It is
thought that sometime soon after the Buddha's enlightenment, divisions
unfolded within the newly created Sangha, with schools of thought developing between 500 and 300 BCE under the broad labels of Mahāsaṅghika

---

5. For more accounts of the formation of contemporary global diasporic communities see
Arjun Appadurai's *Modernity at Large* (1996) and Benedict Anderson's *Imagined Communities*
([1983] 2006).

6. The Sangha can refer to the official Buddhist order of renunciates as well as the more
informal community of Buddhist followers. The Sangha, the *dhamma*, and the Buddha together
constitute what are referred to as the Triple Gems of Buddhism, the cornerstones upon which a
Buddhist practitioner, whether monastic or lay, "takes refuge" and models his or her religious
practice. For summaries of Buddhist teachings passed down through monastic education in Thailand in particular see McDaniel 2008 and Veidlinger 2006. See Cassaniti 2015a for an analysis
of a Buddhist sermon that reveals some of the congruities and incongruities of lay and monastic
relations in Thailand.

and Thera. The Mahāsaṅghika schools eventually became known as the Mahāyāna (the "Great Vehicle") and dispersed into northern and eastern areas of Asia (as well as in Southeast Asia around present-day Thailand). The Sthāvira school of the Thera lineage flourished in Sri Lanka and later also blossomed in mainland Southeast Asia, becoming known by the term "Theravāda" (the "Way of the Elders"), also referred to as Hinayana (or "Small Vehicle") by Mahayanists. It is this branch of Buddhism that dominates the religious landscape of Thailand, Burma, Laos, and Cambodia in mainland Southeast Asia today. Buddhist ideas and practices are transmitted textually and socially in Thailand, especially by monks' teachings and through the Tripitaka, a set of three kinds of texts or "baskets" that make up the Buddhist Pali canon: these are divided into the *suttas* (discourses of the Buddha), *vinaya* (the codes of conduct for monks), and the *Abhidhamma* (discussions of Buddhist psychology).[7] Commentaries and sub-commentaries elaborate further on these teachings, the most popular kind taking the form of *dhamma* books presented with bright colors and a self-help style sold everywhere throughout the country, including at corner convenience stores in remote villages like Mae Jaeng.

While most people agree that Theravada traditions dominate the Buddhist religious landscape in Thailand, religious influences are far from singular, and scholars have long argued about how to best classify the many religious beliefs and practices in the region.[8] Powerful political reforms from governments and royalty over time have contributed to the contemporary religious scene,[9] as have foreign monks and laypeople traveling within Southeast Asia, through networks of Buddhist knowledge that are

7. These three "baskets" of the Tripitaka are usually considered to make up what is called the Theravada Buddhist canon. The edited volume *How Theravada Is Theravada?* (Skilling et al. 2012) and Steven Collins's "On the Very Idea of the Pali Canon" (1990) however raise some important questions about the study of Buddhism as supposedly consolidated into a finite set of texts and ideas.

8. See Hickman 2007, Kitiarsa 2005, and Kirsch 1977 for discussion on the multiplicity of Thai religious practices and the problems of labeling them alternatively as "Theravada," "animist," "syncretic," "hybrid," etc.

9. Politics has always been interwoven into Buddhist practices; governments and the Sangha continue to reinforce and legitimize each other now as in the past. See Keyes 1989 and Jackson 1989, 2003 for some of the historical co-construction of Buddhist practices and Thai politics in Thailand; see McCargo 2004 and Haberkorn 2011 for more recent analyses of political influences in Thai Buddhism.

becoming increasingly global.[10] Non-Theravada regional religious traditions (including those labeled Mahayana and Brahmanic) have helped to
mold contemporary religion, with different lineage teachers and teachings and their accompanying labels interacting historically. Local spirits
called *phi* in Thai have also done so, inhabiting the trees, buildings, and
land throughout the country.[11] All these influences and more are felt in the
religious landscape in Thailand, along with the Theravada teachings of
the Tripitaka. Practices in Thailand with their diverse, personal forms are
summed up no doubt overly neatly by the check box on Thai census takers'
forms that simply say "Buddhist."

In Mae Jaeng religious life is part of the larger social scene. The Mae
Jaeng River snakes through the valley, with a bustling covered market
right next to the bridge over the water in the middle of town, and shops and
services lining the two main streets. Fanning out in all directions beyond
the shops are farming fields with clusters of about fifty houses apiece,
with palm trees and the golden spires of the many monasteries dotting
the landscape. In each direction a few miles farther off tower the green-
covered mountains of the jungle, creating a kind of bowl with the valley
community making up its sloped floor. In the hills around Mae Jaeng lie
ethnically Karen villages,[12] where people practice blends of Buddhism,

---

10. For more on the transnational circulation of Buddhist ideas see Anne Blackburn (forthcoming, on maritime travel between mainland Southeast Asia, India, and Sri Lanka across the
Indian Ocean), Thomas Borchert (on monastic connections between Southern China and mainland Southeast Asia), and Brooke Schedneck (on European and American Buddhist cultural
exchange programs in Thailand).

11. The spiritual landscape in Mae Jaeng is incredibly diverse, but it is usually approached
by people in Mae Jaeng as part of rather than apart from Buddhist thought. Hungry ghosts, for
example, are understood to haunt the living precisely because they are not able to yet let go of
their attachments to the world; the spirits of the mind (locally called *khwan*) similarly are thought
to become out of sorts and cause sickness when one becomes stuck or fixated on something. In
the chapters to come I bring in the activities of the two spirit-doctors (*moh phi*) in Mae Jaeng, for
example, when Mae Daeng gets a cold and when Sen is sick; the spirit doctors prescribed floating away worries in a boat and detaching the spirits of the alcohol as cures. For more on spirits
in Northern Thailand see Johnson 2014; McDaniel 2011; Morris 2000; Formosa 1998; Cassaniti
2015b, Cassaniti and Luhrmann 2014, 2011.

12. The Karen (or Pakinyaw, in the Karen language; Kariang, in Thai) are an ethnic group
distinct from the northern Thai. In the past the Karen were referred to by the term "hill tribe"
and are now thought of as one of Thailand's many "ethnic minorities." The Karen are of Tibeto-
Burman origins, with a unique language, political structure, economic system, cultural system, and
history. Most Karen people live in Burma, but approximately three million call Thailand home,

"animism,"[13] and Christianity. On a dirt path to the west, about fifty kilometers distant, lies the country of Myanmar (Burma), but most people in Mae Jaeng don't travel in that direction. Instead they choose to head east over the mountains to Chiang Mai, the regional capital city, and sometimes travel farther south to the other provinces or the national capital of Bangkok, or even farther abroad to other countries for work and holiday. When my Mae Jaeng friends' grandparents were young they would walk over the mountains for days to get to Chiang Mai, going only when necessary and living on rice and shrimp foraged in the rice fields, and mushrooms and vegetables from the forest. Back then Mae Jaeng was fairly isolated, I was told, known most for itinerant forest monks passing through, and magical monks and opium huts, where officials from Bangkok would come to vacation and indulge in the relaxed upcountry lifestyle. Today a paved road winds up the mountain to Chiang Mai, and the trip takes just two hours. People continue to find food in the rice fields and the forest, but they also drive to Chiang Mai regularly for health care, education (including religious education), and fun, and to replenish their supplies in the big city.

There are about five hundred households and two thousand people in the central valley of Mae Jaeng, and as in virtually all rural areas in Thailand, most of them are farmers. About 65 percent of households farm the

---

among them those living in the areas surrounding Mae Jaeng town. In the district of Mae Jaeng (rather than the center town itself), Karen people make up almost half the population. There are approximately 1.1 million Karen living in 2,132 villages in Northern Thailand, with many more living across the border in Burma. The Karen people in Ban Ko Tao, who are the Karen focus of this book, are S'gaw Karen, the most populous subgroup of Thailand's so-called hill tribe minorities. According to local memory in Ban Ko Tao, the village became Christian about one hundred years ago, missionized by a Karen man traveling from Burma.

13. Over half of the Karen in the area are Christian, with many of the rest following a blend of Buddhism and "animism." The term "animism" as a catch-all "other" category of local spiritual practices carries with it a host of conceptual problems, but it continues to be used at times today to describe religious beliefs and practices centered on the worship of animate spirits residing in inanimate objects. Both Karen and Northern Thai (*kon muang*) people in Mae Jaeng follow forms of "animism" in this sense, but the specifics of beliefs and practices differ from neighborhood to neighborhood. Animism as religious practice was made popular in the work of the early anthropologist James Frazer but is now thought to be a kind of conceptual shortcut describing a range of diverse practices each of which has its own particular and elaborate history and meanings. "Supernaturalism" is sometimes used to relate to some of the same practices, with similar problematic connotations.

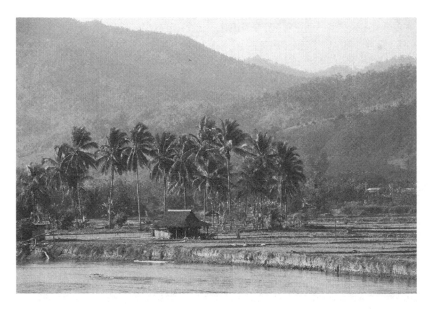

Figure 2. The main valley floor of Mae Jaeng. Farmers plant rice in the valley and live in small neighborhood clusters of villages at the base of the hills. Photo by Rosalyn Hansrisuk.

land in some form, for the most part growing rice in the fields but increasingly growing other crops too, including watercress, peanuts, soybeans, and corn.

Fifteen percent or so of the residents are small-business workers, with stalls at the market or with shops selling goods that they buy in bulk on trips to Chiang Mai. The rest, including some of the farmers and business owners, are *karachagan*—government employees who serve as hospital workers, police, teachers, and town administrators. Most households farm and engage in business of some kind at the same time, growing crops and selling them at their market stall or running a shop and during planting and harvest times working in the fields when they can. About 5 percent of the population in Mae Jaeng is ordained in the Buddhist Sangha at any given time, with the small Buddhist monasteries called *wats* housing on average five to six fairly permanent monks, but with numbers fluctuating from one monk in residence at some of the more remote monasteries in the hills to upward of fifty or more at the novice wat schools or during the annual rainy season retreats.

Religious practice in Mae Jaeng is fairly typical of any rural valley community in Thailand.[14] Each of the small clusters of houses around the valley make up a *moo ban*—a group unit best translated as "village" or "neighborhood"—and in each *moo ban* is a small wat. The wats are a staple of the community and serve as a focal point of social life. People told me that if a neighborhood doesn't have its own wat it is not considered to be a real neighborhood at all. Some wats, like the one in the neighborhood where Goy lives, are thought to have structures over a thousand years old; others are brand new. Virtually everyone visits his or her wat often to make merit, on weekly Buddhist days called *wan phra*, or on special occasions like Asanhabucha (a national holiday celebrating the first sermon of the Buddha) or a *poy luang* (local festivals celebrating the construction of a new monastery building). Formal religious engagement is fairly unstructured; many people stop by their neighborhood monastery regularly whenever they feel like it, whether to visit monks before a big exam, or when someone is ill, when they could use some advice, or just to see friends at events. People visit other neighborhood's wats, too, for ordinations or funerals or festivals. These seem to be happening all the time. As one Mae Jaeng friend told me, "Here in Mae Jaeng we're crazy for wat festivals."

It is a well-known fact in Thailand that the central activity and one of the main goals of religious practice is to make merit. Merit making (called *tham bun*) consists of ritual offerings made to the monks and monastery, and generally of doing things that are considered to be good.[15] There are many other religious activities in addition to this merit making: a central one is that of monastic ordination. Virtually all males, some at a young age, ordain as novice or full monks for a period of time in the Buddhist Sangha to gain merit and practice the *dhamma*. People offer food to monks in the early morning and pay homage to the Buddha through chants at night. Some go on meditation retreats, and many

---

14. This is especially so for the region of Northern Thailand, an area consisting of people and practices under the umbrella term *muang*, a Tai cultural group related to the more politically dominant Tai group of Siamese in Central Thailand. For more on the political and ethnic groups of mainland Southeast Asia see Wijeyewardene 1990, 1984; Davis 1984.

15. The term *tham bun* comes from the Pali word *pun-ya*, for merit, and is based on gaining positive karma. In some ways it is similar to the Sanskrit-based term *puja* in Hinduism. For more

learn about the *dhamma* online. Everyone engages with formal Buddhist activities to some extent.

Religious practices in Mae Jaeng are complex and often draw from multiple historical traditions at once. People float boats and lanterns for religious reasons; they visit spirit doctors for mental health; they offer food to spirits in spirit-houses that are mini-replicas of human homes, placed in front of their real homes; and they make sense of the events in their lives through the Buddhist teachings they grow up with. Most generally this means following the Five Precepts and the other shared religious ideas of the community. These ideas are not always part of the everyday conversations of Buddhist people in Mae Jaeng, but they are very much a part of everyday life.

I had come to Mae Jaeng because I was intrigued about how Buddhist ideas are lived in everyday life—not inside a wat, not abstracted and isolated from the pressures and interests of day-to-day living, but as part of them. Religious life in Mae Jaeng is more than just an engagement with formal Buddhism; it is about a range of emotional and behavioral practices that make up the cultural psychology of people in the community.[16] Most of the Buddhism I had learned before coming to Mae Jaeng was either in books or through meditation trainings at retreats that were purposefully set apart from the everyday. In Mae Jaeng people read books on Buddhist teachings and meditate during retreats at Buddhist wats, but like most Thai people they do neither of these very much. Instead they live Buddhism as part of a taken-for-granted way of being in the world.

Goy told me how, when her father died, she thought about how everything is impermanent, and that she felt better by thinking about it. As I

---

on karma see Doniger O'Flaherty 1980 for a rich analysis of karma in religious texts from South and Southeast Asia, and Keyes and Daniel 1983 for ethnographic accounts of karma in practice in Theravada Buddhist contexts. Also see Cassaniti 2012 for more on explanations of karma and its connections to Buddhist agency and belief in Thailand.

16. Cultural psychology speaks to this emphasis on the relationship between shared cultural ideas and individual mental processes. A subdiscipline of social psychology and cultural anthropology, and closely related to the subdisciplines of cross-cultural psychology and medical anthropology, cultural psychology seeks to "spell out the implicit meanings that give shape to psychological processes, to examining the distribution of those meanings across ethnic groups and temporal-spatial regions of the world, and to identify the manner of their social acquisition" (Shweder et al. 2008, 409). It suggests that cultural ideas and practices are part of (rather than apart from) human

continued my interviews on Buddhism in Mae Jaeng I kept coming back in my mind to these conversations with Goy. How could the idea of impermanence make someone feel better in the face of loss? I decided to learn more about the role of this Buddhist teaching in practice. Attending to impermanence, I realized, means attending to some of the ways that Buddhism is lived in Mae Jaeng.

The Experience of (Studying) Impermanence in Mae Jaeng

I first encountered the concept of *anicca* in Mae Jaeng in an unlikely place. Gaew, another woman around my age I had met in town, owned a store with her parents and brothers near the central intersection of the town, and I had gotten into the habit of stopping by in the afternoons to say hello. I was there with her and with her younger brother Noi, who at eleven years old was about to enter sixth grade, and as usual we were chatting behind the front desk as customers came in and out of the shop. We were looking through Noi's "Society and Buddhism" textbook to prepare him for the upcoming school year and found a passage on the *Trilak*, the idea of the Three Characteristics. It read as follows:

> These rules of nature refer to a state of being that naturally and independently prevails.
>
> They are recognized as common characteristics shared by all things:
>
> 1. Anicca: "impermanence," transience, the state of coming to life and eventually perishing, change.
> 2. Dukkha: "agony"; state of controversy, incompleteness, defect, constant change.
> 3. Anatta: "non-selfhoodness/soulessness, no-self," no real existence of self.[17]

mental processes and examines how this is so for particular people in particular places and times (Shweder and LeVine 1984; Stigler et al. 1990). My emphasis throughout on "practices" rather than "behaviors" or "rituals" reflects the way that people think of their actions as aimed at developing themselves over time. They don't just do religious actions; they practice them.

17. *Sangkomsuksa sasana leh watanatam moh sam* (2551 [in the Thai calendar; 2008 in the English calendar], p. 299), Nantaburi, Thairomklaw, Thailand. The author's translation.

The passage went on to discuss *anicca* at greater length: "*Anicca*, uncertainty. That which arises, must pass away. Instability." *Anicca* seemed to refer not just to physical changes but also mental changes, really to everything one could think of or see or do. The more I learned, the more intrigued I became. While most cultures and religions have some concept of change, Buddhism's emphasis on *anicca* struck me as unusual, if only because it was so marked and elaborated. From what I could tell, non-satisfactoriness is considered a constant, if sometimes low-level, state of existence precisely because people wish for there to be permanence in the world, especially in terms of wishing for a permanent self. But no matter how hard people wish for this to be the case, it just is not so: change is omnipresent. A wish for permanence in the face of change will, according to this teaching, propel suffering because such a wish is impossible to fulfill.

A few months after reading Noi's schoolbook, I stopped by Goy's shop to have some tea. Her aunt came over to tell us a head monk from a nearby village had died, and she invited us to the funeral. Goy and I climbed into the back of her pickup truck, and we drove up a dirt path into the hills, past a school, rice fields, and a picturesque wat to the funeral at the edge of the village. The dirt road ended at a hillside overlooking the mountains around Mae Jaeng. In the middle of the field was a gold coffin topped with flowers. Above it, suspended thirty feet in the air and supported by bamboo poles, was a cloth orange square, symbolizing the community of monks. Hundreds of people were sitting and squatting on the right side on the hillside among the trees, all dressed in black. On the left was a pavilion with about thirty or forty monks in their orange robes and shaved heads.

As Goy and her aunt and I settled into the woods with the others, the monks came forward and put flowers in the gold bowls next to the coffin. Then the men from the hills walked to the coffin and added their flowers to the bowls. Next, the women came and added their flowers; we went with them down to the coffin and held our hands in *wai*, raised with palms together, as we placed onto the coffin the flowers that Goy's aunt had given us to contribute. After we put the flowers down, we went back up to the hill. We sat down, and the announcer began to describe the monk's life:

"Phra Ao Wat was seventy-two. He was born in Phrae Province. He was a police officer for fifteen years, and when he arrived in Mae Jaeng he founded this village wat. Now he has met the end of his life, as we all will have to do." Some men went up to the coffin and removed the big picture of the monk from the site and rearranged the flowers. A monk took the microphone and spoke to the crowd, now in Northern Thai dialect, now in Pali chants. As they prepared to light the coffin on fire, the monk's voice grew more solemn, and I heard the Pali chant a monk had pointed out to me in a book at the library in Wat Pah Ded, one of Mae Jaeng's many wats:

> Alas!
>   Anicca! Impermanent are all things.
>   That which arises is bound to cease.
>   The calming of this is the highest bliss.
>   For a brief time only lives this body, and then it is laid upon the ground,
> consciousness fled; as useless as a rotten log![18]

Soon after a quiet settled in the valley, and then the whizzing sound of a small smoking projectile came out from the pavilion, crossed the field, and set the coffin on fire. Sparks flew 150 or 200 feet up in the air as the fire bullets met the coffin and exploded with loud bangs, trailing smoke below them. Soon the air was smoky and loud, with people squinting in the sun as they moved around. The top of the coffin caught fire first, and soon the whole thing was lit. People's faces were a bit somber but also relaxed, as if they had just spent a casual and fun though weighty afternoon at a picnic. Almost immediately after the fire began everyone started leaving the woods, climbing back onto motorcycles and into the backs of pickup trucks to head home. In the past, I was told, people would return home with their clothes inside out, so that the ghost of the deceased would not be able to recognize them and follow them home. That practice has disappeared, but there remained a kind of quiet rush as people hurried away. I thought about that day long afterward. Unlike funerals in the United States, which typically are modest events mainly for family and friends,

---

18. *Suat Mon Chabap Pak Nua Ruapruam leh Riabriang Doi* Amphur Muang Jangwat Lampang, 2531 [1988].

funerals in Mae Jaeng were well attended by even distant acquaintances. (I myself attended dozens.) The prominence of talk and chanting about impermanence at funerals struck me. There are few moments where the impermanence of living comes to the foreground as much as it does in the case of death, and it was in times of death that the teaching of *anicca* seemed especially prominent—and pertinent. In life, many people can and do try to hold on to a sense of permanence. But at death, the irrevocable truth of change becomes harder to ignore.

I talked with a monk at Wat Pah Ded about the chant I'd heard at the funeral. He showed me a book of funeral chants, of which a prominent one discussed *anicca*. "Alas!" it started out, "Impermanent are all things." As the monk explained to me, this particular phrase is repeated at every funeral in Mae Jaeng, "and as far as I know," he said, "at every funeral throughout Thailand, too." Monks would intone this and many other chants long into the night via loudspeakers while family and friends sat around the coffin, burning incense and talking together until the morning, when the body was then taken to a field and burned.

The more I learned about *anicca*, the more I found evidence of teachings about it in Mae Jaeng. One night I stayed overnight at Gaew's house, and before she turned off the light to sleep she murmured a few lines from a chant book. It was a small book, a leaflet almost, of chants that she like many others in Mae Jaeng read quietly out loud before going to sleep each night. "Dukkha, anicca, anatta," read one of the chants. Teaching about *anicca*, it said: [Nothing is stable. Nothing stays the same. Life is suffering. It is not truly our own]"[19] If found in a book of English-language poetry, such lines could easily be interpreted as despair, or served as a lament or a dirge—yet Gaew read them in almost a relaxed, calm, and casual way. Clearly not just for Goy but also for Gaew and others in Mae Jaeng, being reminded of *anicca* was a good thing; it helped somehow.

A few months later Noi finished his first semester at school and became a novice monk for ten days over his summer vacation. "Ordaining" as a novice monk for a short period was a fairly typical thing to do for kids his age in Mae Jaeng. Noi and ninety-nine of his classmates ordained together—it felt a little bit like summer camp. I went to the ordination

---

19. *Botsuatmon luangputuat watchangpah Jangwat pattan.*

ceremony with Noi and his sister Gaew, his older brother Sen, and his parents Mae San and Paw Nui. We sat in chairs set up around the *vihan* with the other proud relatives. Part of Noi's ordination proceedings, as in all Thai ordinations,[20] included teachings about impermanence. On that first day when I heard these teachings, spoken in a mix of Thai and Pali, I understood only some key terms, like *anicca*, *dukkha*, and *anatta*. Noi and his ninety-nine classmates read from a sheet, which Noi gave me a copy of afterward. One of the chants read as follows:

> Many times He has emphasized:
> body is impermanent,
> feeling is impermanent,
> memory is impermanent,
> volitions are impermanent,
> consciousness is impermanent;
> body is not self,
> feeling is not self,
> memory is not self,
> volitions are not self,
> consciousness is not self;
> all conditioned things are impermanent,
> all dhammas are not self.[21]

Later at a neighbor's house I came across a *dhamma* book lying on a coffee table; in it I read the following, which similarly if more colloquially talked about change:

> This world of living beings that we live in,
> There is nothing that stays.

---

20. The control of all officially recognized Buddhist ordinations in Thailand was established in an edict by the head monarch in Bangkok in 1932 as a nation-building program, giving greater power to the Bangkok-based Thammayut sect, labeling other, rural lineages under an umbrella category of Mahanikai, and streamlining the Thai Sangha. King Mongkut's reforms also made a big impact in the practice of Buddhism in Thailand. This was done in part to modernize the country and consolidate control in the hands of the Thai elite (Kamala 1997).

21. Other than those who study Pali at length, most people in Thailand do not understand very much of the language; the meanings of some common chants become familiar through repetition, while others like this one are spoken in a mix of Thai and Pali to help make sense of the terms,

Nor do people stay.
No one is really the "big person."
There is nothing that belongs to you.
We have to throw everything away.[22]

Together, these experiences convinced me that I needed to have a better understanding of how the concept of *anicca* was understood in Mae Jaeng. According to most scholars, monks follow a form of high Buddhism that incorporates concepts such as *anicca* into chanting and rituals, but these concepts do not reach into the fabric of everyday life. In short, such a perspective suggests, there is a "high" Buddhism as well as a separate, "low" or "village" Buddhism. Was this true? Was *anicca* something that average people thought about only at funerals, when monks told them about it explicitly at the end of loved ones' lives? Was it something they learned only at the wat, during ordinations or meditation retreats? Or was it more meaningful than that, an integral part of a coherent way of thinking about the world? This is not a trivial question, for it goes to the heart of what makes Buddhism matter in people's lives, how they relate psychologically to the ideas so prominent in "high" Buddhist thought.

"Go Ask the Monks"

I drove my motorbike two hours over the hills from Mae Jaeng to Chiang Mai University to speak with Ajarn Somwang, a professor of religion and philosophy who had taken an interest in my research. I was eager to know what a respected scholar of Thai Buddhism thought about my idea that concepts such as *anicca* might be important in the everyday psychological lives of people in Mae Jaeng. When I raised the subject with him,

---

and the meanings of the words of still others remain unrecognized even as they are thought to be powerful or efficacious. The translation of the Pali chant that Noi provided is from the "Ordination Procedure [Upasampadàvidhā] and the Preliminary Duties of a New Bhikkhu," compiled by HRH Supreme Patriarch Somdet Phra Mahà Samaõa Chao Krom Phrayà Vajiraàõavarorasa Mahàmakuñaràjavidyàlaya, translated by Siri Buddhasukh and Phra Khantipàlo (King Mahà Makuta's Academy Bangkok 2516/1973).

22. *Botsuatmon leh kampleh watpasukatoh 20 Tammuthet 4.*

he laughed and told me that "people in the countryside don't know about these difficult teachings about Buddhism. These teachings are part of the literary world of Buddhism, in the Abhidhamma. For regular people, it's not part of their world."

I was surprised by his response, but over time I would come to realize that Professor Somwang's views were far from unusual. Time and again, in conversations with monks and scholars in Thailand and even in the United States, I heard that *anicca* was a part of Buddhism that was outside the everyday. "It's high Buddhism," I would hear. "People in Mae Jaeng wouldn't know about it." As one monk told me, a PhD student at Chiang Mai's Buddhist university of Maha Chulalongkorn Rajavitthayalai at Wat Suan Dok, "*Anicca* is actually the highest teaching. The monks can understand this; the common people don't understand. The monks understand because the monks have more free time for learning. Regular people can't understand, because it is the highest teaching, it is part of philosophy." According to this thinking, either you had to be a scholar (of the formal or "state" Buddhism) or a renouncer (as an ordained monk or as a lay meditator) to take the teaching seriously.

"Countryside folk," in contrast, are seen by scholars to follow a kind of lower level, or superstitious, or "village," or somehow *other* kind of Buddhism, a qualified kind of Thai Buddhism in which people mostly make merit to ask a spiritual power for help, engage in magical beliefs, and accumulate karma to hope for good fortune in present and future lives (McDaniel 2011; Engel and Engel 2010; Kitiarsa 2005; Spiro 1982). Because these practices of merit and magic that people in Mae Jaeng and elsewhere follow are also at times considered to be "not-Buddhist," or at least counter-doctrinal in some way (with ties to Hindu Brahmanism or pre-Buddhist Thai spirits), a "real" or formal Buddhism is often described, if only implicitly in the abstract, as existing somewhere other than in the everyday lives of ordinary Buddhists. This Buddhism may exist in *dhamma* books in Thailand and the West, or in universities, or, if regular people wanted to take the teachings seriously, in meditation centers isolated from everyday life; but they were not seen to occupy a central place in the everyday lives and minds of regular Thai people. I heard that there were two kinds of Buddhism: a Buddhism of the abstract texts and a "popular" Buddhism of the uneducated masses. The people I heard this from, of course, inevitably align themselves with the first kind.[23]

I came across this dichotomy of high vs. low Buddhism not only in conversations but also in scholarly texts. Buddhadasa Bhikkhu, the most famous and influential Thai scholar monk of the past century, railed against what he considered the superstitious practices of the average Thai Buddhist. Phra Payutto, who took up Buddhadasa's mantle as perhaps the most famous Thai scholar monk after the former passed away, echoed the idea. In writing his book on Buddhism, Payutto went as far as to dismiss what most people did and thought: "In explaining the Dhamma," he said, "I will try to show the actual Buddhadhamma that Lord Buddha taught and intended. I will not be considering the popular meanings generally understood by many people, because I feel that they are peripheral and not necessary for understanding the actual Buddhadhamma at all" (1995, 48).[24]

But if the teaching of impermanence is part of a scholarly Buddhism that is too difficult, overly doctrinal, abstract, or unimportant for average Thai Buddhists to follow, why had Goy talked about it so passionately and

---

23. The class issues that undergird much of the supposed division between elite and lay Buddhism are part of Thailand's ongoing political problems. In the minds of many elite Thai Buddhists the religion is split into two versions, with the poor understood to be following an incorrect or flawed version. Political scholar Eli Elinoff has framed it this way: "Elites say, 'The poor are ignorant and can't understand the world they live in [and Buddhism properly] because they have to work all the time. They aren't as well informed as we are.' The poor, rural, and provincial say, 'We understand quite well thank you very much, impermanence is a fact of life when you are at the bottom of late-capitalist Thailand'" (personal communication). For more on the politics of class-based divisions of Buddhism in Thailand see Elinoff 2014; Streckfuss 2011; Gray 1986.

24. In American scholarship the anthropologist Melford Spiro reached a similar conclusion about Buddhism as being a different sort in practice in everyday life in Thailand's neighboring and fellow Theravada Buddhist country, Burma. In his seminal work *Buddhism and Society*, Spiro argued that while ideally a Buddhist would aim for *nibbana*, practicing Buddhist teachings such as those of *anicca*, *dukkha*, and *anatta*, most people he encountered in his fieldwork seemed less interested in nirvana and more interested in accumulating merit (positive karma). Spiro famously went as far as to say that there are different categories of Buddhism, most notably a system of *nibbanic* Buddhism and a system of *kammatic*, with *nibbanic* Buddhism being concerned with release from *samsara*, the wheel of continued existence, and *kammatic* Buddhism concerned with better positioning within it (Spiro 1982). This dichotomy, Spiro says, is prominent in Buddhist countries, and for the most part does not overlap: "Although [the practitioners] don't use these terms, they know precisely how nibbanic differs from kammatic Buddhism, in both aim and technique. If they follow the latter system, it is not from ignorance of the former, nor from a confusion of the two; it is, rather, because they have knowingly chosen the one and rejected the other" (1982, 13).

articulately? Why had I come across it in books at people's homes and at funerals in Mae Jaeng? It may be that those who create culture feed ideals to people that they cannot and do not live by; but my own experiences in Mae Jaeng led me to question this assumption. In fact, I began to wonder if the picture of lived Buddhism painted by scholars and monks was an overreaction to earlier Orientalist scholarship that had assumed an automatic internalization of Buddhist teachings and missed the nuances of what it meant to live ideas in practice. Having seen for myself signs of greater engagement with *anicca* in Mae Jaeng, I decided to go to the source and ask people directly about it.

"Do you know the Buddhist teaching of *anicca*?" I asked people around me in Mae Jaeng. "How is it influential in your day-to-day life?"

"Oh," I would get as a response, "I don't know about *that*. That's difficult, abstract teaching. Go ask the monks about it." I was surprised again! It seemed I was wrong: the responses seemed consistent not with my hypothesis of knowledge and interest about impermanence but rather with the assumption of an uninformed, uninterested layperson.

After a few similar responses, I decided to take people's advice and go ask the monks to explain *anicca* to me. I went to the wat in Ban Hai, the village I was living in on the edge of the Mae Jaeng valley. Novice monks were running around when I entered the wat grounds, scrambling to smooth out their robes when they saw me, while trying to pretend they had not just been in the middle of a soccer game when I showed up. "Could you tell me a little bit about *anicca*, the Buddhist teaching of impermanence?" I asked the older, more senior monks when I sat down with them a few minutes later for an interview.

"Oh," the head monk replied, almost echoing the lay responses, "we don't know about *that*. This is a small, rural wat. We're just trying to feed and house these boys. Go talk to monks in Bangkok about this."

It seemed I was wrong again. Faced with the same demurring response from monks as from laypeople, I felt puzzled. It is not that monks in Mae Jaeng did not know about *anicca*: I had heard them talking about it in sermons. The idea that I would be referred to the scholar monks in Bangkok points to the same problem I had had with laypeople: the monk was referencing an imagined (and politically real) hierarchy of a particular kind of Buddhist knowledge. This knowledge is the kind represented in textbooks and formal Buddhist philosophy. The conclusion that not only laypeople but also ordained people felt unable or ill-equipped to talk about *anicca* suggests a kind of Buddhist orthodoxy or elite control, the same kind that many scholars take for granted when they choose to focus on the voices of "experts" for their research. Except in the case of certain laypeople meeting certain life situations, like Goy, there was a view that it was separate from everyday living.

I discussed what I had learned with Goy. She impressed me as different from many of the others I had spoken to, and more open to talking about abstract ideas. I asked her to tell me more about *anicca*. But at first she told me, surprisingly, the same response as everyone else: "The technical terms of *anicca*, *anatta*, I don't know them. You should ask the monks." As a graduate of Chiang Mai's Payap University, Goy was more educated than most people and had shown a clear and elaborate interest in *anicca* when I had first met her; I had expected her to readily offer elaborate views on the subject, but she seemed reluctant when I asked explicitly, perhaps because it was thought to be the domain of the ordained. She said: "I know a little, though, like that *anicca* is about the impermanence of life. The monks taught us. You have to know it yourself. Who are you? Where do you come from? Not—Julia from USA—our parents make us human, but before that, we don't know—you have to study yourself." It almost seemed as if she had to show some deference to the monks, to the official, formal hierarchy of Buddhist learning, before starting in on a topic she had already in the past discussed at length. When I asked her for advice on how to get people to talk about *anicca*, if they did have anything to say, she suggested talking about *anicca* more personally, rather than as an abstract teaching, to ask people about it in a way they could relate to.

Goy's insights proved prescient. I returned to asking people about their Buddhist practices rather than *anicca*, about what might be called rituals or routines, as I had been doing and had been trained to do, but I continued to include a question or two about change at the end of the discussions. I introduced more colloquial words to talk about it, too. Rather than (or in addition to) the Pali term that by its ties to the revered language of Buddhism marked it as part of formal discourse, I introduced different terms: Thai phrases like *khuam mai nae non* (uncertainty); *mai tiang* (instability); and *plien pleng* (change).

Initially, for the most part, I got the same responses: "Go to the wat and see the monk. The monk will explain. I don't know anything about that." As I talked with more people, though, and became more comfortable in the community, I noticed a different discourse starting to unfold. After professing an almost complete lack of knowledge about *anicca*, some people told me stories about it, little anecdotes to illustrate the teaching, almost as asides. One woman, after telling me that she knew nothing about *anicca*, seemed to mark that the formal interview was over and moved away from the mat we had been sitting on and onto a weaving stool. There, as she started to weave, she continued talking about a topic she had just said she didn't know anything about: "The impermanence means that you do everything, like wage labor, to get a lot of money—but you don't get a lot of money. You do farming and earn a little, sometimes you lose. Sometimes we expect a large income from farming, but then we get only a small income. You have a good yield but the price is low. . . . We always lose in farming. Impermanence is when you want or need something but you can't get it. Don't think about it anymore."

A farmer told me, "Yeah, we have experience with impermanence— every year in farming in Mae Jaeng! Some years you make a profit, some years you lose. Don't have high expectations. Impermanence means we can't expect the price for the harvest for next year to be good. It's better to think of the chance as just fifty-fifty." Another farmer said, "Like when I've lost something. For example, suppose the land is damaged or flooded, we feel sorrow. Or the thing we most love, we feel sorrow when we've lost it. The idea of impermanence means we want to take something, but we have to stop our need. When I think of impermanence I feel better."

Finally, I was on to something. These farmers talked about impermanence not in terms of an abstract fact of life but rather in the tangible reality of their lives. It was not only farmers that talked about change; businesspeople in Mae Jaeng did as well. One woman, a successful weaver who sent her woven cloths to be sold in upscale markets in Bangkok, told me, "I don't make high expectations in my business. I keep some part of my mind without hope because of impermanence. If things don't work out, I want to be OK. Don't have too large expectations, because something may happen at any time." And another business owner, who was less successful, voiced a similar perspective: "If my business is good it's good for me; if my business is bad I try not to feel sad. This is *anicca*. What shall I do? I can't do anything. I can only think of innovations for selling things, and try again next time." People *do*, it turned out, incorporate teachings of impermanence into their everyday lives, and draw upon them in a way that reflected a sophisticated understanding of impermanence and its role in Buddhist thought.

Once I stopped asking about it, and started instead to listen for it, talk about impermanence seemed to be everywhere. Talk often included didactic statements. People invoked *anicca* for what seemed to be the purpose of self-work, advising themselves to temper their emotional reaction to a catastrophic event, or even to temper the emotions against the mere possibility that such a catastrophe might occur. *Anicca*, whether an external idea worked into the self, or an already given orientation toward events, was very much present in people's minds. So why had I heard that people would not know about *anicca* in a rural place like Mae Jaeng?

The answer to this difficult question has to do with the personal nature of the teaching and the ways it relates to shared discourses of power and religiosity in today's Thailand. Rather than evoking a discussion of an abstract fact of life tied to other abstract facts of life like *dukkha*, *anatta*, the Four Noble Truths, or the Eightfold Path, when I asked about *anicca* in Mae Jaeng I was told that while the teaching had first been heard at the wat, it was only really learned through everyday experience. People may have formally heard about it in a book or at a monastery, but the lessons and understandings about it, I was told, came from outside these frameworks. As such, there was little formal knowledge, but a high degree of informal understanding. As one somewhat exceptional monk in Mae Jaeng told me, in an unusually frank conversation,

> Everyone thinks about *anicca* in their lives. They think about it all the time, maybe when they get up in the morning, and before they go out. The people here, they understand. They know, but they don't know how to explain about *anicca*. If the person is a teacher it is their job, they can explain, but not the common people in the field. I think everybody thinks the same about impermanence, more or less. They get this understanding from the wat and from their experience in real life. From the wat they learn the preaching and teaching of the *dhamma*, but *dhamma* is nature. We can apply our understandings from life.[25]

While that monk had been talking for the most part about laypeople, he and other monks I spoke with voiced similar attitudes. Monks couched

---

25. It might be possible that it is the older and adult generations that think about (elaborate, emphasize, understand, or feel) impermanence more. "Kids don't think about it," one old man told me, ". . . because they're kids." Another told me, "I think about it more as I get older." "Yeah, my mother-in-law thinks about *anicca* more than I do," one man told me one afternoon while I was

their awareness of impermanence in their own personal interests: in addition to talking about *dhamma* books they had read and lessons they had heard, they told me about the impermanence of monkhood itself, in the form of friends who leave the monkhood or leave to stay at wats in different towns; they told me about the impermanence of their physical body, which they told me they saw from watching their hair and nails growing; they told me about the change that had happened to their lives once they ordained. The head monk of one of Mae Jaeng's many wats reiterated the idea that learning about impermanence was a personal project. "You have to know yourself," he told me, "know and understand life. People do not all have the same idea of *anicca*. Don't compare it with science."[26]

---

explaining my project, "but that's because she's older. When I'm in my fifties I'll pay attention to it as much as she does." Another woman, in her fifties, told me the same about her mother, who was learning about *anicca* and other aspects of Buddhist philosophy at the *wat*, where she had started sleeping at night.

26. This advice seemed to counter almost directly the way Buddhism was taught in universities and in popular books; in those contexts, Buddhism was very much likened to science, as a rational philosophical project. The idea of Buddhism as rational and scientific has a long history and helps to explain the dichotomy of abstract and lived Buddhism so often presented in Buddhist studies scholarship. Scholars often quote a passage of the Buddha's teaching that discusses shirt-sleeves: "Look," the Buddha said, rolling up his shirt to the elbow, "I have nothing up my sleeve." The idea was that everything he said could be, and should be, encountered through direct experience. In this sense, the words I heard in Mae Jaeng about learning about *anicca* through experience were similar to the idea the Buddha advocated. But this emphasis on experience, along with other teachings likening the Buddha to a "medicine man," suggested a "scientific" outlook that became a cornerstone of Buddhism over time. Philip Almond, in *The British Discovery of Buddhism* (1988), traces the emergence of Western scholarship on Buddhism at the end of the nineteenth century and the beginning of the twentieth. Almond argues that certain wishes of these scholars for a rational philosophical Buddhism (led by Rhys Davids and the Pali Text society, along with similar wishes by governments and royalty [especially King Mongkut] in Thailand, to display, or create a "state-sponsored" Buddhism that was scientific and rational to counter colonial attitudes of "backward" nations) created the kind of dichotomy that I had encountered when speaking with people in Mae Jaeng. (See also Thongchai Winichakul's *Siam Mapped* [1994] for a historical construction of modern Buddhism in Thailand.) When anthropologists and travelers began to document Buddhist practices in the mid- and late twentieth century they found that Buddhism "on the ground" did not fit neatly with the rationalized and "scientific" accounts that the religion has become famous for. It was this disjunction, in part, that caused a second wave of observers to reject the overarching abstracted and rationalist representation by which Buddhism had come to be known, and to begin to claim that people in the countryside follow a second, less abstract system of Buddhism called "*kammatic* Buddhism" or "village Buddhism." In this perspective Buddhism in practice was to be understood as centrally about things like superstition, merit making, and ritual, and that abstract ideas like impermanence, nonself, and suffering are part of a higher philosophical realm in which people living everyday lives in Thailand take no substantial part.

These monks were like the others in applying impermanence to personal experience, rather than treating it as a realm of knowledge apart from the everyday.

"When I Think of Impermanence I Feel Better"

The concept of *anicca*, clearly, is alive and well in Mae Jaeng. I wrote about my findings after that first summer in Mac Jacng (Cassaniti 2006) and figured I had made inroads into understanding how Buddhism is lived in Northern Thailand. And yet a thought kept nagging at me: people told me that thinking about *anicca* helped them feel better; but why? And how? Why would thinking about impermanence make someone feel better? Had I answered that? After all, Goy had told me that after her father died and she started learning more about impermanence, she had started to feel better. She said her brother Ta didn't learn much about impermanence or become interested in Buddhism; he went to Chiang Mai and fell in with a bad crowd. He had started taking opium, she told me; he was still suffering from the family's loss.

In Noi's ordination proceedings, after relaying the different aspects of life that are impermanent and without self, the chant had continued:

All of us beset by birth, decay and death,
  by sorrow, lamentation, pain, grief and despair,
  by dukkha, obstructed by dukkha,
  |consider| that it is well if the
  complete ending of the dukkha-
  groups might be known.

Why is it "well" to know about *anicca*, as this Buddhist chant suggests? What is it about *anicca* and well-being, even mental health, in Mae Jaeng? When I looked over the notes from my interviews about *anicca* I noticed that many of them seemed to be about emotion: "If my business is bad I try not to feel sad."

When I had first become interested in *anicca* I had expected people in Mae Jaeng, if they talked about it at all, to talk about it in a way similar to what I had heard from scholars and monks and scholarly books: *anicca* is an abstract fact of life that relates to change, to suffering and not-self, and that an awareness of it results in the lessening of suffering. When people I talked with did not discuss the term in this abstract way, I had thought they were unfamiliar with it, or only superficially understood it. When I did manage to get people to talk about impermanence, they spoke in a tone that was different from what I had expected to hear. Not only were the discussions personal, connected to personal interests, but they also often took on an emotional tone. *Anicca* seemed not only to explain events but to offer something to help people emotionally.

One of my last days in Mae Jaeng in the summer of 2002, I opened my eyes in the morning to see a strange face staring at me, waiting for me to wake up. It was an old local woman, and she spoke to me excitedly in the Northern Thai dialect that I was still learning. "They died last night!" she said. "They were on a motorcycle, and they crashed!" She was telling me this, I found out later, because one of the people who had died was a foreigner, and as few foreigners visit that part of Thailand, she assumed I knew him. I didn't, but I did know the other person on the motorcycle. He was Anurak, the uncle of my friend Gaew, and after a late night of drinking at his karaoke shop with his new foreign friend they drove home at 4 a.m. and somehow ended up in a ditch.

I went to the funeral that morning at Wat Gu, Gaew's neighborhood wat. Gaew and Noi and Sen were there, their faces wan. They and their family did not portray overt displays of anything that looked like sadness, even though ten years later they still spoke with fondness of Gaew's uncle. Gaew talked to me about how she was scared of his ghost. She also told me, as a way to help herself and also make me feel better, that we never know what will happen. Nothing is certain. Everything is impermanent. The general affect in the wat was one of quiet calm and reserve, even to such a sudden, shocking, violent death. I was struck by the calmness at the funeral. While I didn't foresee it then, I would get to know Gaew and her family much better in the years that followed and would come to realize that this calmness was a central part of ceremonies and conversations about a wide range of big and small events.

A few days after Anurak's funeral I was in the nearby city of Chiang Mai at a motorcycle rental shop returning the motorcycle that I had rented for the summer. The owner there, "Mr. Beer," mentioned that a westerner had died in Mae Jaeng that week. The westerner had rented his motorcycle from the same shop, and Mr. Beer brought me to a back room where

I looked at a mangled, contorted Honda bike much like the one I had just returned. "They returned the bike to me," the owner said, "but I don't know what to do with the guy's passport he'd left for me while he had it." He paused, then went on, "I guess he doesn't need it anymore." I thought of *anicca*, of uncertainty and impermanence, but thinking about impermanence did nothing to help me feel better. I felt awful. If I felt anything from thinking about it, I felt a bit sad, and depressed. Certainly not comforted.

Anthropologists have noted an apparent lack of sadness or "grief" after death in Thai communities, but have attributed it to a subduing of displays and suppressed expression of emotion, thereby suggesting that grief is felt but somehow "kept inside" (Keyes 1983). I didn't get that sense from Goy when she talked about her father, or from Gaew at her uncle's funeral, or from the many others I have gotten to know since then. I didn't get the sense that people's feelings of calmness in the face of loss are the result of suppression; it was much more complicated than that.

Metaphysical ideas of Buddhism are not always part of the everyday conversations of Buddhist people in Mae Jaeng. But they are very much a part of everyday lives. Emotions, attachments, and the effects of intentional action (more popularly called karma) are felt in personal stories and events and show that, like *anicca*, real life doesn't always neatly fit into formal boxes of Buddhist teachings. Everyone has his or her own interpretations and experiences; but through this diversity a shared perspective emerges that helps to answer the question that Goy pointed to when she first talked about her father's death, and that Gaew pointed out when her uncle died. People feel better by thinking of impermanence because it reminds them that getting stuck on things will bring suffering. By crafting calm and "cool-hearted" emotions, the inverse suggests, one is able to more easily let go of affective attachments, creating positive results.

Positive and negative examples of calmness and cool-hearted emotion point to moralized affective orientations for people in Mae Jaeng, and are my concerns in the first two chapters here. Affective attachments to objects and people highlight practices of letting go, and struggles unfold through holding on to these attachments; they are my focus in chapters 3 and 4. The final chapter is on karma, reflected through the meeting of past action and future results in the present, and serving as a system of moral causal action on the effects of emotional attachments. Together personal engagements with impermanence, emotion, attachment, and karma work to craft health and well-being. To relate this I draw from observations and conversations with Goy, Gaew, Sen, and the many others I got to know over the years in Mae Jaeng. Throughout I examine rituals at the wat, discussing how people interpret them, and for comparative contrast to practices in Mae Jaeng show how ideas and practices about emotion, attachment, and causality differ in a nearby but culturally distinct Karen Christian community. In the beginning I lay out some of the more structured methods I followed in conducting ethnographically oriented interviews, and over the course of the text I make increasing use of close relationships with members of the community to illustrate the personal, felt complexities that engaging with Buddhist ideals entail, especially through an increasingly close account of Sen and his struggles. Throughout I show how emotion, attachment, and karma work together in Mae Jaeng. Such practices reveal a side of Buddhism that is real and lived, not just confined to historical texts or abstract ideals. It shows how people are living Buddhism as part of the culturally complicated psychology of everyday life.

Part I

EMOTION

1

Cool Hearts

Goy's family spread through Mae Jaeng, from the family's house behind a wat near the center of town, out to the market down the road to the main town intersection, and across the bridge over the Mae Jaeng River. The river meanders slowly through the valley, swamping the fields in the rainy season and lying low for people to build bamboo huts over to relax by in the dry season. It floats across the valley floor and continues on to the regional capital of Chiang Mai, following a long path through the mountains, eventually making its way to the Chao Phraya River in Bangkok and finally out to the Gulf of Thailand. The dust in Mae Jaeng doesn't make it as far: it accumulates, turning the few paved roads into mud when the rain comes and rising again as thick dust in the heat. On the sides of the roads are shops and houses, most of them wooden but with a few concrete ones for the bank, the hospital, and a few new stores. Every five hundred meters or so are the serpent statues marking the entrance to a wat, the golden spires of the buildings reaching up farther than the houses and the palm trees around them and creating a sparkling glean to the landscape.

When I returned to Mae Jaeng for a year of extended fieldwork, Goy invited me to stay with her and her mother Mae Daeng at their house, and I happily moved in. Mae Daeng's nine brothers and sisters all lived in Mae Jaeng, with extended relatives staying at the family outpost house in Chiang Mai or farther away, even to the United States where her niece Niw worked as a nurse in Baltimore, Maryland. When I first arrived, though, all I saw of this family network was a large house at the back of a larger compound on a side street at the edge of town, backed up to the post office and the neighborhood monastery of Wat Ko. Mae Daeng had a vegetable garden and an outdoor kitchen, and in the evenings a seemingly never-ending cycle of friends and family would gather to grill pork and vegetables and eat in front of the fire for a few hours, the same fire Goy's father had died in front of the year before I had first come to Mae Jaeng.

Mae Daeng was smallish, round, and cheerful compared to her daughter's tall, quiet demeanor. She talked nonstop in the Northern Thai dialect, *kam muang*, about whatever was on her mind. Mae Daeng and I got along well, though we didn't always understand each other, and not just because of language difficulty. The first day I moved into the house, Mae Daeng showed me to my room and said, "When Goy's friends come to visit from Bangkok they can stay in here with you too and share the bed with you."

I was taken aback at the prospective loss of the little vestige of privacy I had thought I would have. I recalled the anthropologist Jean Briggs's ethnographic account of living in a tent with an Inuit family for a year, and the struggles she had in trying to maintain her own space (Briggs 1970). I figured I had to take a stand early to avoid problems later: "No . . ." I told Mae Daeng, as definitively as I could while still being mindful of the fact that I was the recipient of someone else's hospitality. Neither Mae Daeng nor Goy had asked for money for my stay, laughing and telling me I was their daughter and sister when I had offered and saying I could help out here and there by bringing home vegetables for dinner or doing little things around the house instead. I didn't want to seem territorial in the face of their kindness, but I also didn't want to share a room. "I need my own space," I went on, "just for me. With a lock on the door when I'm out and no one else coming in." She agreed, but was perplexed.

That night she stopped by the doorway to my room again in her nightgown. "Don't forget to take a shower before you go to bed," she told me.

"I'm OK," I replied. "I took one this morning, and I haven't moved around a lot, so I don't need to take one tonight."

Mae Daeng and I looked at each other for a moment, and she smiled uncertainly and said good night. No one in Thailand avoids taking showers at night. Months later, skipping an evening shower would come to seem almost unthinkable, but at the time the two of us gazed at each other curiously across the door of my room as if from two different worlds.

Goy and her mother had an easy camaraderie, with Goy making most of the decisions in the household. They came and went, a bit like room mates who cared about each other and happened to be related. Unlike the instant bond I forged with Goy, her mother and I took time to grow on each other. Soon, however, we were inseparable. On outings to the wat or to events around town she had me accompany her everywhere, almost like a pet. Goy was glad—I later realized she had invited me to stay at her house partly to keep Mae Daeng company while she was at work and her brother was away in the city—and her mother and I were glad too. Mae Daeng's constant comments on the people and events around her filled up my field notes, and provided a much-needed sense of support and security in what was still a strange place to me.

In the evenings, Goy and Mae Daeng and I would, like most people, find our way home from the fields to sit for dinner in the front of the house. Throughout Mae Jaeng, families sit outside, grouped on mats eating dinner: spicy vegetable dishes and fish with sticky rice and sometimes *lao*, the local rice whiskey. By 9 p.m. it's bedtime, and all the lights in town go out under the luminous expanse of the night sky. In the early morning, while it was still dark, Mae Daeng would head out to the canopied local market down the road by the river, where she and about fifty other vendors sell vegetables and other goods at their market stalls. Vendors line the bridge across the river as early as 4 a.m., while the moon is still out and the morning still quiet, spreading out their goods across their mats. People living in the villages up in the hills come down to town at this time, too, to buy goods to take back for the day. Customers from the hills were mostly ethnic Karen, but there were also members of the Hmong, Lahu, and Lisu communities; they crowded into the market area, with embroidered local dress and their own histories and languages. Everyone seemed to be up early; even Aung, a friend of Gaew and Sen who liked bright makeup and went to party at the discos in Chiang Mai when she could, woke up well before dawn every morning to slaughter the pigs she had raised in the shed behind her house, and bring them to the market to sell before the sun rose.

I on the other hand slept in almost every morning, waking up at what I later learned was the audaciously late hour of 7 a.m. "Especially for women," Gaew's brother Sen told me, laughing, "they should be awake really early." Mae Daeng would stop by the house around eight to take a break from her work at the market and cook Goy and me some vegetarian *nam prik*, a spicy Northern Thai dish of vegetables and chilis from the family garden and sticky rice from the fields. Goy and I ate breakfast together if we were around at the same time, and talked about how her business was going at the stationery store, or about the traditional Northern Thai children's music group she was putting together to promote Northern Thai culture, or her work as a DJ for Mae Jaeng's local radio station, or my experience getting to know people around town. After breakfast Goy would go to her store or to garden at her plot of land. Sometimes she would head back to the shed behind her house and get on the airwaves to broadcast the radio program she ran, playing traditional Northern Thai music interrupted occasionally with news and comments on community events.[1] I would leave for the day, too, after breakfast, mostly at first just to wander around and talk to people and get to know the area. I spent a lot of time exploring Mae Jaeng, chatting with neighbors and looking around the village and fields at the edges of town, where groups of neighbors would take turns planting and harvesting one another's land. At the fields of people I knew I sometimes joined in, my back starting to ache almost immediately from bending in the sun to plant little bunches of rice plants in the watery field, but more often I would find a hut in the field instead, where the farmers sit for breaks from the midday, to sit down in and read. In the huts at midday, everyone opened dishes of food that had been prepared at home, lounged and chatted for a bit about the land and their families. I would join them, or would sit alone at an empty hut and read books about Buddhism. I read about theories of karma and dependent origination, set out in abstract phrases that seemed to refer to another time and place.

Sometimes a farmer would stop by, surprised to see a foreigner on his or her land, and even more surprised that I spoke Thai. We would then

---

1. I discuss Goy's position as a unique kind of modern traditionalist in "The Rural DJ," part of the edited collection *Figures of Southeast Asian Modernity* (Cassaniti 2014b).

proceed to talk about farming for a while before he or she would walk away with a machete in hand to continue with work in the fields. By the early afternoon I would have returned to town for lunch at the *som tam* (papaya salad) stand near home. This started as a solitary ritual, but as time went by I would take my meal to Gaew and her brother Sen's shop house to share with them. Gaew and Sen lived a few hundred meters from the main intersection of town, in a two-story place with three storefront sections open to the street. The siblings Gaew, Sen, and Noi, along with Gaew's husband Pan and their parents Mae San and Paw Nui, all lived upstairs from the shop. The shop sold everyday goods, from cosmetics to snacks, and served as a kind of gathering place for friends and neighbors around town. I spent most afternoons at the shop working on my Thai language skills with Gaew or Sen, teaching them English in exchange. At first I tried to make sense of the system involved in the operation of the store, but I quickly realized it was run informally: Gaew, Sen, or their mom or dad would work the counter, often for a few hours at a time, until one of them would stop by to say "I've got this now," or "Go get something to eat," and take over. Sometimes Noi would sit with them, though at eleven years old he wasn't quite ready to manage the desk himself. I would sit on the bench next to Gaew or Sen, chatting with customers and doing as they did, putting things in bags and handing out change, unloading ice from the delivery truck or going to get drinking water from the natural well. The family atmosphere was casual, jocular, quiet, and relaxed. Gaew was chatty and friendly, while Sen was more reserved, with a charismatic smile that I came to look forward to seeing. He drank while we were out at night, but while I was getting to know him in those early days he seemed fine. In the evenings I returned home to have dinner and watch what the royal family was up to that day on television with Mae Daeng, who liked to watch the nationally broadcast royal family show when she wasn't out at a monastery event around town.

Special occasions came up often around town, usually in association with a Buddhist event of some sort. Once a week, Mae Daeng went to her neighborhood's wat, Wat Ko, around the corner from our house, for *wan phra* (in Northern Thai *wan sil*), the weekly "Buddha day," where she and our neighbors made offerings and paid respects to the monks near the thousand-year-old stupa while they chatted and socialized. It seemed like festivals of some kind or another were always taking place: for the building of a new monastery, a merit-making fund-raising festival for some

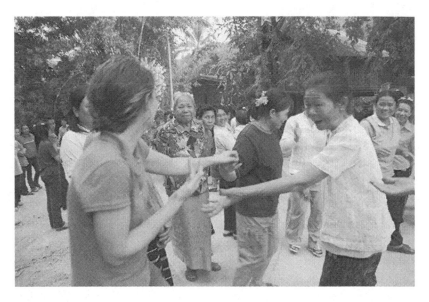

Figure 3. A wat festival parade; the author is being invited to participate as local women dance on their way to the monastery. Photo by Rosalyn Hansrisuk.

community project, an ordination, funeral, sporting event, or some other national or local holiday. Mae Daeng and her friends would sit listening to monks, practicing rituals like pouring popped rice into bowls of incense, tying white strings at Buddhist ceremonies, or proceeding through town in dancing, often drunken parades.

I wanted to know about Buddhism and its influence on Goy, Mae Daeng, Gaew, Sen, and the others I was getting to know. I wanted to know about emotion especially, because emotion seemed to be implicated in talk about *anicca*. But from learning about *anicca* I realized that it wouldn't work to just expect people to articulate Buddhist ideas and ideals in abstraction, nor to assume if people didn't articulate them that way that the ideas were not relevant for them. Real life is, of course, much more complex.

I was hesitant to push for a certain way of talking or seeing things in the people around me. Instead of jumping into interviews or talking about Buddhism explicitly I just generally hung around early on, participating in and observing local practices. I played ping-pong and bocce ball ("the queen's favorite sport!") with Mae Daeng's young niece Wan, Wan's mother P'Dao, and others at the side of the river at dusk, continuing to play until what seemed to be late into the night. I laughed with them when they stated their disbelief that a government agency called the Fulbright Foundation from my home country was actually paying me to be there and play games with them. I got to know people and people's gossip; I got to know that Goy was considered unusual in her serious outlook on Buddhist teachings ("If Goy were a man," I overheard Gaew whispering to her friend Aung one afternoon, as Goy's voice on the radio announced another wat festival, ". . . she'd be a head monk!"). I got to know that Mae Daeng's twin sister Mae U lived in a "bad part of town," even though that part of town was only a few hundred meters down the road and seemed to me to be virtually the same as Mae Daeng's neighborhood. I learned about more interpersonal gossip than I could keep up with in my journals, including neighbors' romantic escapades (the man across the street from Gaew's got his mistress pregnant and was now living with her *and* his wife!); I learned about relatives' adventures, and the sordid details of acquaintances' lives. I listened and explored as much as possible, scribbling in my notebook by day and typing up the scribbling into field notes at night. To learn more I started volunteering at the local branch of Thai Rak, an environmental NGO from Bangkok, and teaching English to novice monks at Wat Pah Ded, one of Mae Jaeng's three monastery schools that the novice monks from the other wats in the valley would attend. For the most part, though, I worked at getting used to the pace and tone of life in the community.

I wanted drama, the kind that seemed "anthropological" somehow, with conflict, tension, striking rituals of magic or healing, rowdy festivals or fights. I wanted the Balinese cockfights of Geertz (1973a), the superstitions of Malinowski's Trobriand Islanders (1922), or the headhunting and rage of Rosaldo's depictions in the Philippines (1984). But nothing much seemed to happen. There were a lot of rituals and festivals, and I went to as many as I could and wrote about them all in my notebook, but there didn't seem to be much in the way of emotional encounters or outpourings of feelings. People didn't seem to get angry, or sad, or full of joy, or excited, as far as I could tell. I didn't encounter these or any of the other emotions that, as I had been taught in my psychology classes, were universal and cross-culturally basic to human experience. On television the news from Bangkok sometimes showed people riled up about the latest political scandal, but it was looked at by people around me literally as if from another country.[2] According to the *Oxford English Dictionary*, emotion is "any agitation or disturbance of mind, feeling, passion; any vehement or excited mental state." But aside from little flickers here and there of what that might be, I couldn't find much in the way of agitations or disturbances at all.

Jai Yen: Calmness

I wanted drama, but everyone seemed so calm. One evening as I was talking with Goy over dinner, she told me about a cloth-weaving festival that would take place in Mae Jaeng the following month. The annual festival drew Thai tourists from as far away as Isaan (Northeastern Thailand) and Bangkok, and culminated in a parade through town with representatives from the different ethnic groups in the valley and hills showing off their finest clothes. I knew how much Goy liked traditional Northern Thai culture, and how much she liked to be involved in local community events, so I said to her, "I'm guessing you're involved in planning this?"

Goy paused and said, "Well, you're right . . . it's something I'm interested in—I went to a planning meeting last week. But they want to sell the clothes, and make it a marketable business event. They say, this way, villagers will be more likely to weave cloth garments and banners for the festival and participate in it, and that selling their clothes will inspire more pride in their craft . . . but I disagree. I think selling the weaving at the festival is

---

2. Historically the region of Northern Thailand has been made up of its own regional kingdoms that have been in different degrees at odds with surrounding regions, including that of present-day Central Thailand (Penth 2000). Even today Central Thailand, the seat of the Kingdom of Thailand's present administrative center, is thought of as a kind of separate country by most Northern Thai people in Mae Jaeng. Politics in Central Thailand are felt in Mae Jaeng; over the course of just two years, from the beginning of my extended fieldwork in 2005 to a return visit in 2008, "Red Shirt" support for the exiled prime minister Thaksin Shinawatra went from just one woman in town to almost everyone. This regional tension is felt in everyday religious practices as much as in political identifications. For more on the historical carving out of the political and cultural territory of Northern Thailand see Winichakul 1994; Keyes 1995; and Penth 2000.

a bad idea; the weavers will become distanced from their craft and see it as an object for money, instead of having real pride in the tradition."

"So what did you say to them? What happened?" I asked, ready to hear about a rousing debate between Goy and the others at the meeting.

Goy laughed, "Nothing. I left."

Goy seemed fine with the outcome of the meeting; she seemed calm and comfortable with it. The next week she put on a traditional Northern Thai dance performance at the local wat, and talked about it on the radio show she DJ'd, and moved on from the cloth festival.

Early one morning Mae Daeng brought me to the government building at the main intersection of Mae Jaeng to make merit by offering food to the monks. The monks lined up to receive our food in the parking lot as the sun rose for another one of the town-sponsored merit-making festivals. There were a lot of people out and about, even though it was only 6 a.m. I followed Mae Daeng as she put a small bundle of toiletries into each bowl. The mood was quiet. I saw Gaew there, and she came up to me:

"Julia, I thought you were meeting me to go to the wat this morning. I waited for you."

"Oh no, I totally forgot," I replied, flustered, as I remembered the plan I'd made with her the day before. I was worried that she would be annoyed. "I'm sorry!"

She looked at me and laughed, "*Mai pen rai* [never mind], it's OK!" She wasn't upset, as I supposed she would be.

Moments of cool-heartedness were everywhere. I was sitting chatting quietly with Gaew another afternoon at the shop in the center of town when a man entered to buy some goods. "Two bottles of whiskey, five sodas, and twenty baht of ice," he said, pointing to the icebox for Gaew or me to retrieve his order from.

I started to quickly put together his order, and he told me to slow down: "*Jai yen*," he said, smiling.

"*Jai yen*," I repeated back to him, smiling and relaxing. I was starting to train myself in the local lexicon of emotion.

The calmness of a cool heart in Mae Jaeng is captured in this phrase *jai yen*, and the cool heart of a *jai yen* is everywhere. The Thai word *jai* literally means the heart, or, according to one Thai-English dictionary, reflects a complex of "the heart, mind, spirit; spiritual center or core; soul; inner being."[3] There are hundreds of Thai compound words with the term *jai* in them, and the most common *jai* expression is *jai yen*, literally a "cool heart."

Sometimes when I stopped by Gaew's shop for our afternoon language exchange I found that she was not quite ready to begin, and I would say "I'm ready—let's start our lesson!" but in response she would tell me the same thing I was hearing from others: to wait and be patient. "Julia, *jai yen yen*!"

Only on rare occasions did someone act in the unattractive way called a *jai ron*, a "hot" or "impatient" heart, waiting in line at a food stall while the server was too busy chatting with a friend to attend to her customer, or crowded in on the pickup-truck taxis that drove people over the mountain to Chiang Mai and back. In those instances I would invariably hear their neighbor or friend say to them, laughing, "Jai yen yen na"—"be cool-hearted," or "be cool."

When I look at my field notes I'm surprised at how many times I wrote casually about people being calm, even when I didn't expect them to be.

"Mae Daeng's sister is out on the street, talking in a high pitch, looking for Ta (her small son), but she's relaxed," I wrote. When Goy's cousin Jip ordained as a monk for a few months before becoming a police

---

3. This definition is from http://www.thai-language.com. In Thailand the heart is seen as a seat for feelings that range in disposition and heat in hundreds of different ways. Like the gut, the liver, and other bodily sites used in different cultural contexts around the world to describe the location of feelings, the *jai* in Thai works as the central idiom for linguistically couching emotion in the body. The English language draws a similar attention to the heart as the place of feeling, but the set of compound *jai* words ranges in scope well beyond English notions of the heart and extends to realms considered in English to reference not only affective but also cognitive states, dispositions, attitudes, and even actions. There are hundreds of ways to describe the feelings of the heart. A Thai–English language book called *Heart Talk* lists more than seven hundred *jai* terms in use in Thailand (Moore 2006), and while some of these terms seem to point more to cognition than emotion, all are part of what American scholars would call an emotional lexicon. Along with *tham jai* and *jai yen*, one can feel *kreng jai* (deferential), *jai dii* (friendly), *jai ron* (hot and impatient), *jing jai* (persuading), *khow jai* (understanding), *nam jai* (helpful). The list goes on and on, but a "cool heart" of *jai yen* is the most popular. A bilingual Thai language teacher in Chiang Mai years ago once summed up nicely in English when I asked whether *jai yen* is a feeling. She said, "Anything with the term *jai* in it relates to feelings."

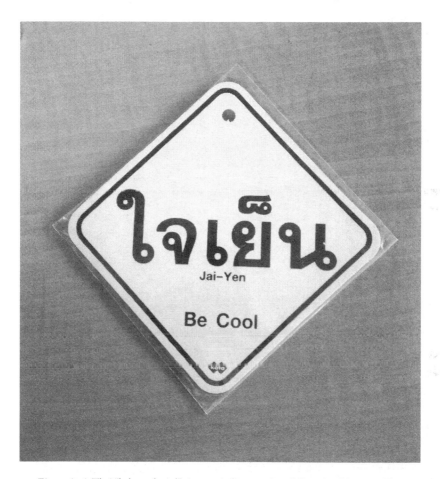

Figure 4. A Thai "baby on board" sign reminding people to follow the ubiquitous Thai emotional orientation to *"jai yen"*—be cool.

officer, I described the event in my notes as boisterous, but also somehow still calm:

> In front of the house Goy and a bunch of people are playing musical instruments. I look at Jip: he seems a bit apprehensive, but mostly calm. Everyone is playing music, and it's starting to get louder. We head out into the quiet street, down the main road and across the bridge. There are about fifty people, it's about 8:30 at night and already most of the houses around us

are dark . . . it feels peaceful and calm, even with the noise and the parade. After it's over we go back to get our bikes, Mae hurrying a little ahead of me because it's started to rain. The next morning they do the *namo tassa* and 3 *buddham dhammam saranam gachami* chants [basic Pali Buddhist chants] and other ones. The head monk holds a fan in front of his face as he speaks. Mae Daeng's trying not to yawn: "underneath the fan here it's cool and easy to be sleepy," she says to me, smiling sheepishly. There are about ten or so lay men sitting toward the front, and then the women about thirty behind them. Two monks come out and chant quietly, perfectly in time with each other. It starts to rain.

In the early months when I still didn't know many people in the community, I sat at home with Mae Daeng often in the mornings and the afternoons, and as often as not she would turn to me and say, "Julia, let's go to the wat. Wat Ban Tap is having an ordination ceremony today." Or, "At Wat Gu there's a merit-making festival."[4] Or, "I have to drop something off at Wat Pah Ded for a friend, let's go." Sometimes when I would get home at the late hour of 9 p.m. I wouldn't find Mae Daeng at home at all, and I would call her and she would tell me she was at a wat: "There's a ceremony here at Wat Jiang," or "There's a funeral at Wat Buddhaen, I'll be back later," and she would show up later wearing a local *tin jok* skirt or a black lacy Northern Thai–style outfit. The next morning she would get up a little later to go to her market stall. When she took me with her to an event, she would help me put my own Northern Thai *tin jok* outfit on correctly, and we would add flowers in our hair before the two of us set out on our way. Sometimes Goy would be at the event, too, usually organizing people sitting around or with a microphone in her hand, to direct people to parking spots or places to put their bright *pha pa* (in Northern Thai

---

4. Making merit is popular throughout Thailand; it may be the most popular and common religious ritual in the country. Merit is positive karma; by making merit one makes positive karma for future use. In Mae Jaeng, merit making is especially ubiquitous; everyone seems to be making merit all the time. Every morning people make merit outside their homes when they offer food to monks out on their rounds; they make merit at the wat on the weekly *wan phra* "Buddha days"; they line up at the front of the town's administrative offices on governmentally designated Buddhist holidays; they make merit when they make offerings to the wat and monks in organized neighborhood "merit-making festivals" on auspicious days, or in a Northern Thai festival called Poy Luang when a new monastery building is made; or as part of an ordination or before a trip, or for a sick friend, or before a big exam in school; or really whenever they feel like it. It's not just at the monastery that people make merit; they make merit when they do anything good.

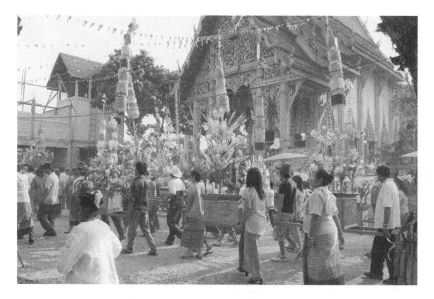

Figure 5. A monastery festival.

tan salak)—handmade "money tree" structures decorated with flowers and bills for making merit.

Beginning the Interviews

When I noticed situations where people were calm or upset I wrote it down, and when in passing I heard someone reference a cool heart I wrote that down, too. The calmness felt different from what I was used to in my life in America, where people seem to rush from one thing to the next. I started to pay more attention to the ways that people seemed calm when I thought they wouldn't be, and to attend to the situation around the moment. Soon, though, the presence of calmness faded into the taken-for-granted, invisible background of everyday life in the community.

I decided to start interviews, which I had planned to do all along but had wanted to hold off on until I had a better sense of people in the community. In chatting between neighbors, in ordination into monkhood, and in daily life in general, the calmness of a *jai yen* had seemed to be everywhere, but I didn't know how pervasive it was in personal lives, or how it was thought about, and when. Goy, Mae Daeng, Gaew, Sen, and their families and friends were all engaging daily with the complex issues of their lives, but for their different reasons these were the people who chose to talk to me. To get a more general, broader sense of the psychology of everyday life in the community, as a complement to the depth of these personal relationships I needed to learn from a larger, more representative sample. I wanted to learn about the ideas of strangers in their homes and work and rice fields in Mae Jaeng, not just the activists, students, artists, or otherwise somehow always slightly idiosyncratic people drawn to and by the foreign anthropologist.

I developed interview questions, mostly open-ended ones that I had formulated from discussions with Goy, Gaew, Sen, and others, to get people to talk about change in their lives. The questions probed broadly for personal feelings and explanations, and ended with more pointed inquiries about religion. Here is a list of all eighteen of the final interview questions:

1. Could you tell me a little about what you were like as a child? How have you changed or stayed the same since that time?

2. Could you tell me a little about a sibling (or close friend)? How have they changed or stayed the same since then?

3. How has this area changed in the last fifteen years? Do you think life was better then or now?

4. Do you remember the recent Southeast Asian tsunami [that had occurred in 2004]? How did you feel when you heard about it? Why do you think it may have happened? (*And after initial responses, other possibilities were offered in a list culled from earlier conversations, with the interviewee asked if any of them made sense.*) Was it because of being a part of nature? Was it because a divine being was punishing those there? Because of bad karma? Because of bad luck?

5. Can you tell me about some time recently when you were surprised by something, when something happened that you didn't foresee? How did you feel about the event?

6. I've heard they're introducing life insurance into this area. What do you think about life insurance? Do you like the idea?

7. Do you remember some instance where you or someone you know lost or found money? Can you tell me a little about it? How did you feel then? How do you feel about it now?

8. Have you ever known or do you know someone who got into a motorbike or other vehicle accident? Why do you think you or they got into this accident? (*After initial responses, other possibilities were raised in a list culled from earlier conversations, and the interviewee was asked if any of them made sense.*) Because the driver wasn't concentrating? Because they were drunk? The driver wasn't being careful? Wasn't driving well? Bad luck? Bad karma? A divine being decided it? Was it *khraw* [a theory of something like fate connected by people in Mae Jaeng to Hinduism]?

9. Have you had a person close to you die recently? Could you tell me a little about that? Why did it happen? When? How did you feel? Why did the person die?

10. Can you tell me a bit about your thoughts on the future? What do you think the area here in Mae Jaeng will be like in fifteen years? What do you think your life will be like in fifteen years? Do you think life will be better than it is now?

11. Of the three ages of twenty, forty, and sixty, at which age do people have the most, least, and middle amount of happiness? Why?

Religion:

12. What is your religion?[5] Could you tell me a little about it, and your experience with your religion? What kinds of things do you do as part of your religion?

13. Do you feel like you follow religion very strongly, or not very strongly? How many times a month do you go to the wat? How many times a month do you *wai phra* [a ritual act that can take the form of holding one's hands together in a "*wai*," or kneeling before

---

5. I was often asked during the course of my fieldwork about my own religious affiliations, and after first trying to avoid the question in the hope of getting more "objective" responses, I soon realized that such a (non)presentation of self was impossible. I was usually assumed to be Christian because I was American, and some people wanted clarification or elaboration. In the first interviews, when I was asked about my religious identity I answered, "I don't follow any one religion," but people seemed aghast at that response. After a few times of watching their discomfort, and after hearing people say that "all religions teach one to be a good person," I changed my response to, "Well, I like all religions. . . ," and most people seemed to be put at ease.

a Buddhist altar and bowing, or chanting *dhamma* texts, or just generally paying homage to the Buddha]?

14. In what areas of your life does religion have a lot of influence? Outside the wat, in your everyday life, when do you think about religion?

15. When you go to make merit or *wai phra*, why do you do these
things?

16. What do you think will happen to you after you die?

17. Have you ever heard of *anicca*, of impermanence? Can you tell me
about it? Where did you hear about it?

18. Do you have any questions or things you would like to discuss
further?[6]

With the questions in hand I decided to find a research assistant to
help before beginning the interviews. I knew Thai already, so the assistant
wouldn't need to speak English, but it would be useful to have another person to work with. Finding a good research assistant was not a task I wanted
to take lightly; many of my friends and colleagues had found people to
help them who had either overly shaped the interviewees' thoughts or else
worked rotely without becoming involved in the unfolding conversation
at all. After I had talked with a few people who didn't seem like a great fit
because of conflicting schedules or a lack of the skills I was looking for, Goy
suggested a local man named Ari Lisa Chuchuhnjitsakul, who had written
a book on local practices for his master's thesis at Chiang Mai University
(Chuchuhnjitsakul 2004), and who now ran a boardinghouse/orphanage
outside of town for children coming from remote villages to stay in while
they attended school in town. Ari was smart, Goy said; he knew people in
the area, and would be able to introduce me to a lot of them. He was also
familiar with social science research. I drove on my motorbike out to Ari's
orphanage, about forty kilometers north on the edges of Mae Jaeng District.
The way was a pockmarked old paved road leading through Karen and

---

6. In addition to the above questions, at the end of the interviews I also asked a series of hypo-
thetical probability questions aimed at gauging ideas about change and its presence in people's
personalities and everyday activities (from Miller 1984, Nisbett 2003, and Ji, Peng, and Nisbett
2000), along with some psychological measures designed to rate ideas about internal and external
locus of control (from Rotter 1966). None of these probes bore consistent or useful data, most likely
because of the limitations of their own cultural construction, so I have not included them in the
discussion here.

Hmong villages on the side, and long expanses of rolling hills lining the way to Mae Hong Son Province at the border of Burma. It was September, the rainy season, and the land was a vibrant green, with rain clouds and a rainbow off in the distance. When I got to the orphanage after an hour's travel Ari wasn't home. After leaving notes asking him to call me I finally connected with him, and we arranged a time to meet.

"It sounds great," he said, "but I'm so busy with the kids, I'm not sure I can do it. . . ."

After some convincing he agreed to help, on the condition that the time for interviewing was flexible and worked around his schedule with the school.

A native to Mae Jaeng and ethnically Karen, the minority group that lives in the hills surrounding town, Ari not only was well versed in the kind of methodological work I needed help with, but also was familiar with the social landscape that I was still getting to know. He didn't know English at all but was fluent in the three main languages spoken in the area: Thai, Karen, and Northern Thai (called *kam muang*, officially a "dialect" of the official Central Thai of the country but considered another language by Northern Thai speakers). My ability to speak, write, and read in Thai had improved dramatically since I first arrived in Mae Jaeng, but to make sure I understood the interview responses as much as possible, Ari would be able to explain more difficult words to me from the interviews using easier ones. He also had a truck, a beat-up old Toyota that alternated between the jobs of bringing schoolchildren into town and transporting buffalo; the truck would prove useful for going out to the neighborhoods in the hills, where the paths up into the mountains were dirt and almost impossible to climb on a motorbike. Together Ari and I worked to translate the interviews into Thai, making copies at the shop across from Gaew and Sen's store. We discussed whom to interview first and decided on Goy's aunt P'Dao, who lives in the house next to Goy in the family compound.

Every morning P'Dao woke up early to stand out on the street as the sun was rising, waiting in the light mist to offer food to the monks. She knew all the monks well, as they were local to Mae Jaeng and stayed at our neighborhood wat. She had invited me to make an offering with her one early morning, and together we had stood at the corner of our compound as the monks came by on their regular morning *bintabaht* (alms round).

After placing the food into their bowls we kneeled as they recited a blessing in Pali, a chant called Bot Suat Sap Pi. Neither of us knew the meanings of all the Pali words spoken, but the chant felt rhythmic and soothing, and we recognized a few words here and there, among them *sati*—mindfulness— and *anitchang*—impermanence. I felt comfortable enough to ask her the sometimes strange and unusual questions on the list, but wasn't so close to her as to fear she would wander too far off topic or laugh at the questions' rather abstract phrasing.

We sat down one afternoon at P'Dao's workplace at the central administration office of town and went through the interview questions.

When asked why she made offerings to the monks, she said, almost off-handedly, "I do it because it feels good. . . . I work hard during the day and don't get to go to the wat a lot, so it's a way to give something, to not think of myself and getting money all the time. I feel good when I make offerings, *yen jai.*"

P'Dao talked about a lot of things that morning, including the health of her older sister, who was in the hospital, and the time she won the lottery, and the time she lost her wallet, and her thoughts on the future of her town. Afterward P'Dao went back to work, and Ari and I walked to a shop by the side of the road to listen to the interview again on the audiotape and discuss what she had said as I translated and transcribed it into my computer. After this first successful interview, Ari and I agreed to meet in the mornings after breakfast at Gaew's shop and take our motorbikes or his pickup truck to find new people to talk to. We decided to interview people in a village outside of Mae Jaeng as well as in town, to get a sense of life in an even more rural area, and picked a hamlet called Chang Kao, about thirty kilometers north of Mae Jaeng down a long dirt road into the jungle at the base of an outlying hill.

A few days each week we stopped in at homes where people were sitting outside and asked if we could talk with them for an hour or so about their thoughts and feelings about their lives and their town and religion. Overwhelmingly people said yes, usually continuing, as we talked, to shuck tamarind shells, watch TV, weave baskets, keep an eye on babies, or whatever they had been doing when we showed up.

We brought snacks to share that we had picked up from Gaew and Sen's shop that morning, which were promptly eaten by the children who were usually surrounding us. Children, friends, and relatives were interested in the tape recorder, the questions, my skin tone, and the thoughts

TABLE 1. Demographic information of people interviewed in two Buddhist neighborhoods: Mae Jaeng town and the outlying Mae Jaeng neighborhood of Chang Kao

	Mae Jaeng town	Chang Kao
Religion	Buddhist	Buddhist
Setting	Main town	Very rural village 30 km from Mae Jaeng
Number of people interviewed	30	30
Average age	42	52
Male / female	M 15 / F 15	M 16 / F 14
Average schooling	2nd year high school (~age 15)	4th year elementary school (~age 9)

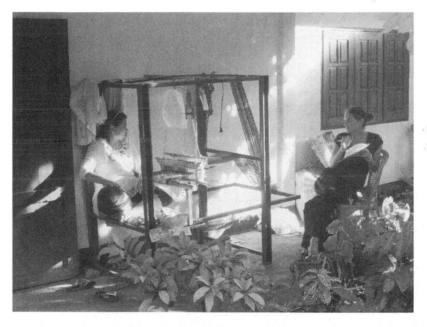

Figure 6. The author interviewing a woman in Mae Jaeng at her loom.
Photo by Rebecca Hall.

their family member was sharing that they probably hadn't heard before. Usually we interviewed people who didn't seem busy, but sometimes we stopped people on their way to or from working in the fields, and with their boots and broad hats for the sun they would sit down with us in a shady spot and talk.

Ari and I interviewed two or three people every second or third day, depending on Ari's schedule with the boardinghouse, sometimes picking up truckloads of schoolchildren or buffalo to deliver on the way, and at the end of each interview we gave each person a thank-you note with fifty baht (about $1.50). Most people laughed at the money and said it wasn't necessary at all, and when we insisted that it was just a token of thanks they took it, most saying they would donate the money to their neighborhood wat. We filled the tape recorder with people's thoughts and feelings, recording them in Thai, Northern Thai, or a mix of the two according to the speaker's preference. After the official interview we would stay to chat some more or head out to find someone else, or if it was late afternoon by that point we would return to Mae Jaeng so that Ari could get his schoolkids with his pickup truck at the end of the day to take back to the orphanage outside town.

The day following each interview Ari and I would sit down in an empty room at his boardinghouse or somewhere quiet in town and go over his notes and mine, listening to the taped recordings as I typed in English. For a whole day we transcribed and translated the interviews of the day before, Ari clarifying points that were complex or new to me, like the backstory of a spirit named Phi Mok who lived in the region, or a political scandal that happened years ago but whose repercussions were still felt, and we would discuss nuances of meanings and tones in the discussions.[7]

Not surprisingly, in all the interviews *jai yen* was mentioned at least once, in connection with feelings about events or as descriptions of friends, family, and self.

My sister, she's got a cool heart. Always has. She's quiet, and calm, and cool.

My brother is someone with a very cool heart, he has a good heart. He doesn't speak strongly.

He speaks well. She has a cool heart, a good mood. She's *sabai*—comfortable.

---

7. Some friends and colleagues I knew had collected taped interviews in their anthropological fieldwork and returned to their home countries without translating or transcribing them, only to find themselves with hundreds of hours of audiotape, no one to help with the transcription, and a fading recollection of the context of the conversations. I wanted to turn every interview into written English as I went along to avoid this possibility.

I'm cool hearted, the same as my sister. I have sympathy for animals, for people. I'm relaxed, I take it easy.

I've got a cool heart. I don't think too much. I'm not easily angered.

Mae Jaeng's current police chief, the man who had taken over when Goy's father died, also used the idiom of a cool heart to describe himself: "I've got a good disposition," he said. "I have a cool heart, quiet and calm. I'm *jai yen*; I see what's around me."

The Monastery as a Site for Emotional Practice

The calmness of a *jai yen* isn't an explicitly religious feeling, consigned only to the space of monasteries and doctrinal texts. But most of the people interviewed talked about calmness in some relation to religious activities. They did not talk about it explicitly as a religious edict, with phrases like "Buddhism says to be calm and cool-hearted," but there was a general sense that cultivating calmness is a good Buddhist thing to do. As the Thai Buddhist scholar Charles Keyes says: "As Buddhists, [Thai] villagers consciously seek to eliminate the 'impurities' of the mind, a value that is usually expressed in village terms with reference to the ideal of maintaining a 'cool heart' [*jai yen*]" (1985, 160). People talked about it as feelings they had when they took part in religious activities. The most explicit of these is the training of a monk. One man told me, "My mind became more peaceful, and calmer, and cooler after I was a monk." Living away from the hustle and bustle of household life, he said, let him take time to study teachings on how to be calm, to practice the always-present meditation of everyday activities of wat life. Even without the mental and physical resources provided by living at the monastery full time, visiting the wat offers a place for people in the community to cultivate calmness.

Calmness in Mae Jaeng is especially marked in monastery settings, but monastery settings can be thought of as part of, rather than separate from, the everyday lives of people in the area. Religious and royal leaders in Thailand have long attempted to centralize and isolate ordained monks from the rest of society as part of a "modernization" project for the Thai Sangha, but in rural communities like Mae Jaeng the monastery and the town continue to be very much intertwined. Young novice monks live in the wat of their neighborhood, and their families visit often. Monks are brothers and sons of everyone, and they often listen to their relatives in planning and carrying out activities like the construction of new monastery buildings and holding wat festivals. Unlike in countries such as Sri Lanka, where monks ordain for life, in Thailand, since the reforms of King Rama VI, monkhood for most is a temporary project, and virtually all males have ordained at least once, often for an extended period before marriage. The wats in Mae Jaeng are on a constantly refilling cycle, with some monks derobing and others moving on to the Buddhist universities in Chiang Mai. The wats are far from empty or distant symbols of religious ideals: they are the social centers of the community and are involved in most of the town's social occasions. People in Mae Jaeng sometimes go to meditation retreats outside of town, remaining away from everyday life in stints that can last from a few days to a few weeks. But seated and silent meditation is not the central part of religious engagement in everyday life, as it is sometimes portrayed to be in foreign accounts of Buddhism. Instead people attend their local wats and incorporate Buddhist practices into hundreds of different kinds of activities; especially during the town's many wat festivals and religious days, the grounds are overflowing.[8]

At wat festivals the monastery is loud, as people greet each other and chat, laughing and smiling. There is a feeling of excitement. But even in this social space, and especially in the *wihan*, the central assembly hall of the wat, there is a feeling of calmness. Inside the *wihan* Mae Daeng shows me how to sit in the back with her friends, mostly older middle-aged women, all of us laypeople facing the Buddha statue and the monks, who also sit on the floor and lead the chants. From ceremonies held before dawn, like the Ha Ping to celebrate the harvest, to ceremonies held all through the night, like the Buk Net celebrating the opening of the eyes of the Buddha (statue) in a new monastery building, to the weekly *wan phra* days when the dawn

---

8. The prominence of the wat in everyday life in Mae Jaeng is juxtaposed with increasing popular public discourse both in Thailand and the United States about Thailand's emptying Buddhist spaces. The decrease in monk ordination in Thailand in general has been linked to both increased accessibility to government secular schools and to an increasingly secular society, but in the comparatively poorer and more traditional area of Mae Jaeng this trend was not found. Although I did notice changes in the ways that people identify with their religious traditions, as they became more personally engaged with the Buddhist teachings and less reliant on particular monks as teachers, it is possible that the decrease in religiosity in Thailand has been exaggerated by popular media.

hours are full of people walking home, to the daylong neighborhood merit-making festivals, nationally celebrated events to commemorate days in the Buddhist calendar, ordination ceremonies, dance performances, and personal merit-making visits to the wat, ritual religious activities are part of everyday life in Mae Jaeng.

I thought that as an anthropologist I would still want to go to these events long after the people who introduced them to me would tire of them. I was wrong. At least once a week Mae Daeng or Goy would wake me up in the early morning and take me to a wat event, or in the evening call to tell me they were at one and to come on over. I would go to find Goy helping to cut paper flowers for decorations or corralling people together, or see Mae Daeng sitting surrounded by her middle-aged friends preparing food, or sitting by a fan in one of the pavilions lining the monastery grounds. The wat is a place people always look forward to visiting and serves as a site for learning about and instantiating ideals in practice. The anthropologist of religion Saba Mahmood makes this point at a broader level, showing how daily rituals can work to determine a certain kind of personhood (Mahmood 2005). By practicing and repeating certain kinds of bodily and affective comportment, people at the wat work to shape their subjectivity by their actions.[9] While this kind of practical "training" is often explicit for monks and other religious renouncers (Cook 2010), its bodily emphasis is less overt but still part of religious practice for everyday lay (non-ordained) people. Most people in Mae Jaeng simply enjoy making wat activities part of their lives. By sitting in *wai* and making offerings, in attending the wat and participating in religious activities around it, in subtle ways a concentrated focus on calmness helps to cultivate embodied affective orientations.

When people talk about engaging in religious activities in Mae Jaeng they use a phrase that means "to practice": *bhatibat tham*, literally "to practice the dharma." Each of the ubiquitous wats in Mae Jaeng has its

---

9. Scholarship on the subject of religious embodiment suggests that particular bodily and sensory forms of training craft culturally varied forms of religious experience (Mauss 1934; Csordas 1994; Hirshkind 2009; Turner 1969). The term "asceticism" itself derives from a Greek term referring to the bodily and mental practices of athletes training to embody certain kinds of subjectivities. Ritual practices in Mae Jaeng that emphasize the letting go of affective attachments reflect such an ascetic orientation to embodiment.

own teachings and lineage, and each serves a slightly different purpose.[10] But one of the most common reasons that people throughout Mae Jaeng attend their wat has to do with cultivating, or practicing, cool-heartedness. When I asked people why they went to the wat and participated in religious activities, the most popular response was to "make merit" (which will be discussed in the following chapters); but the second most popular answer was to feel cool-hearted. The wat and its teachings, even if one thinks about such things when home at night, chanting before sleeping rather than actually at the monastery, or when making an offering to a Buddhist shrine, serve as a site for practicing calmness. When people were asked in interviews directly about reasons for going to the monastery, the cultivation and practice of calmness was cited in over half of them:

> I go to cool my heart and not be like a monkey, like monkeys running around in trees; to not have a life like a monkey; to be quiet, and peaceful.

> When I feel stressed I go to make my heart calm and cool.

> I go to practice concentration, and to have a peaceful, calm heart.

> I sit in meditation and have a cool heart. My mood gets cooler.

> I don't know how my karma is. I go to not have problems or be scared, to make my heart comfortable and calm.

The monastery serves as a quiet place to practice, whether this takes the form of sitting in meditation, making merit, or chatting with friends. At first the explanations of calmness that people offered seemed to be a presentation of a certain kind of self, one performed in interviews to the visiting anthropologist, as much as if not more than a reflection of "real" reasons. After all, it seemed that Mae Daeng went to our neighborhood wat for social

---

10. Wat Pah Ded is an excellent example of the kind of constructive clash of imagined modernity and imagined past found in many sites throughout Thailand. The monastery served for many years as a center for the Thai social activist Sulak Sivaraksa, who promotes a Buddhist-informed socialism and considers that ideal to exist in Mae Jaeng. Ajarn Witti, professor of traditional Northern Thai art at Chiang Mai University, similarly reconceptualized the old as new as old again when he designed the *bot* (ordination hall) for Wat Pah Ded's monastery using new artistic ideas to play with older Northern Thai aesthetic forms. All the other monasteries in Mae Jaeng similarly have their own narratives that mix ancient and recent historical memory. As Goy told me, an excellent history book could be written on each of them.

purposes of seeing friends and relaxing with friends, rather than solely for affective aspirations or ultimate religious goals. When I had directly asked Mae Daeng why she went, her official answer was vague: "Well, I go because it feels good." Goy went to the wat mostly for the traditional community activities; Gaew went usually to *krap* (pay respect to the monks and the Buddha), make an offering, and after five minutes return home. Sen never went to the monastery, but the rest of the family did, and behaved similarly to Gaew. But even as everyone I knew had his or her own personal reasons for visiting the monastery, for many, practicing having a calm heart was one of them, and I noticed it in their demeanor as much as in their talk.

When Noi ordained as a novice for two weeks, he and the other ninety-nine boys who ordained with him spent a night at each of the valley's wats, receiving training from senior monks in a kind of rotating monastic camp. When it was his group's turn to stay at the wat behind our house, Mae Daeng came into my room in the evening and said, "Let's go see Noi at the wat!" I wasn't sure what to expect. After all, Noi was only eleven years old. He was a quiet kid who for the most part seemed to be paid little attention to at his home and was often seen as too young to know much at all. But now he was a novice monk, worthy of great respect, and I wasn't sure how to act around him. I imagined I would feel a sense of somber awkwardness when I entered the wat, but that wasn't the case.

"I don't really know how to act in front of the novice monk Noi," I told Mae Daeng as we walked in. The area outside the *vihan* was lit with candles, and at night the orange robes the boys wore and their shiny, newly shaven heads glowed against the old monastery walls they were sitting against in a line.

She laughed, "Never mind, don't worry about it."

From far away it seemed like a somber, ethereal scene, but close up family members were chatting as they handed out mugs of Ovaltine to the boys. Noi and the other novices looked a bit uncomfortable, like they weren't quite sure how to act, but they were the only ones who seemed that way. Mae Daeng and the other mothers and a few fathers went about talking with each other as if it were any other ceremony that didn't directly involve their children. After wishing Noi well, we headed back home. Back at the house we didn't talk about what Noi's training would do for him, but the ubiquitous feeling of "cool-heartedness" and a religious role in its development lingered from the monastery to the home.

2

HEAT

Goy announced out of the blue one day that her brother Ta would be returning from Chiang Mai to live in our house. Ta had been serving in the army in the city for the past two years and had visited in his military uniform a few times in the past months, but this would be the first time in years that he would be living at home. Goy told me about his arrival a bit apprehensively. "Julia, he's . . ." she tilted her head from side to side, "he's a bit *ting-tong*: crazy. Not *ba*: really crazy. Just . . . off." She seemed a little bit nervous. He moved in without fanfare and seemed nice, deferential to his sister and mother, but after living with him for a few months I agreed: he was a bit *ting-tong*. There was nothing obvious about him that seemed to suggest he was "off," but his demeanor and the way he participated in conversations was often strange; he would speak off-topic or exit the conversation abruptly. His aunt Lah pulled me aside and told me that Ta's oddnesses were the result of his drug use a few years earlier; "then when [Prime Minister] Thaksin [Shinawatra] cracked down on drugs," she told me, "he had to stop taking them; but he's never been the same." After he crashed several motorcycles his license was revoked and he was forced to get around town on foot or by bicycle, the typical mode of transportation in Mae Jaeng for those who suffered from poverty or mental instability.

From the time he entered our household Ta spent his days at home watching music videos on TV, or trying to repair old machines, like a pop-corn maker in the front yard that he dredged up from somewhere, or a wheelbarrow he decided to restore. Sometimes he helped out his mom at her stall at the market, or was sent off periodically to help Mae Daeng's twin Mae U with her shop; but he did no consistent actual work that I could see. He stomped around the house, and he told his mom long elaborate stories that I couldn't follow, and she couldn't either. But although Ta was clearly abnormal in some fashion, he never yelled in the house or became visibly upset.

Ta seemed oblivious of the normally quiet demeanor around him. I had been pulled aside by Goy early on in my stay at the house, apparently after clomping around too much; she instructed me how to move correctly. "Walk quietly, like this," she said, demonstrating how to put the ball of my foot down on the floor before the heel and take quiet steps. I had changed from what I considered a regular gait to this new style almost immediately, but Ta never did, and I could tell his physical style bothered his mother. Sometimes at night Mae Daeng and I would be sitting in front of the television, watching the news of the royal family or some soap opera, and Ta would come storming out of his room to get something from the kitchen. He would laugh at something only he was thinking of, or interrupt people and speak incoherently about politics or pop music.

Not Quite Fitting In

"Be quiet in the house," his mother told Ta as he pounded through while we were watching TV, but he ignored her. "Why do I live like this?" she said, turning to me. "My parents had nine children, they all lived under the same roof, and they never had any problems like this." The way that she dealt with Ta, though, was never to yell at him. Nor did she gather her mental resources to have a big talk with him about his behavior. Instead she worked on maintaining a sense of calm, walking away from him, telling him quietly to stop whatever was bothering her, or just letting him be.

With metaphors revolving around the heat of the heart—a hot heart, a cool heart—so common in Mae Jaeng, tensions in the construction of a cool heart can show what kinds of emotions are especially prevalent and valued in the community. Instances where people didn't fit in with the ideal emotional orientation of coolness (among them Ta, me, children, and those in a nearby Karen Christian community) help make sense of emotion in Mae Jaeng by demonstrating how affect is constructed in practice.

Goy dealt with Ta much the same way that Mae Daeng did, but with a little bit less patience. One day we were outside the house moving a *tuu* (a wardrobe) from Goy's pickup truck to the living room. "Ta, come help," Goy had called out to him in his room, where he had been watching TV. He appeared at the door and tried to help, but Goy gave him too many instructions, and after failing to clear the doorway with the wardrobe, he just dropped it and left. I could tell he was upset at Goy, whom he no doubt considered bossy; I had felt the same way about her at times. But he didn't react by becoming angry; he just left. I looked at Goy's face to see what she would do. She had a blank look for a second, as if she was thinking about something; but then it was normal again, and we resumed our work as before.

Like Ta I also had problems in the house because of my not quite fitting in. In the first few months of my stay I did everything with Mae Daeng, but after a while the interviews began and I became more involved with other things in town. More and more often Mae Daeng wanted to watch TV with me, or go to a wat or just spend a quiet evening at home, and I would leave the house and not come home until late.

"Julia, why do you have to go out?" she would ask at 8 p.m., or "It's late, why don't you stay in?" as I was heading out the door. Goy often did not come home until after 10, and I figured it was acceptable if I did the same. When I explained that I had started volunteering at an environmental organization in town, and that they could only hold meetings after the members had worked at their regular jobs all day, she had agreed. I knew she didn't particularly like it, but I went ahead, only a little bit worried about crossing a boundary of some kind.

One day, about four months into my stay, I pushed a house rule too far—a rule Mae Daeng had apparently set for me without my knowing it. I had taken my motorcycle to visit a nearby village in the afternoon at the beginning of the rainy season, and on my way home, around dusk, it had started to rain, and I stopped by the side of the road to wait out the storm; then I visited Gaew and Sen for a while. When the rain stopped, at around ten, I came home, but, unusually, the house was locked, and I had to knock and wake up Mae Daeng to be let in.

The next morning at breakfast Mae Daeng came over to talk with me: "You come home too late. You don't respect the rules. We don't think you should stay here anymore. We don't think you belong here."

I was crestfallen. "Mae," I asked her, trying to keep my composure, "what did I do wrong? Why didn't you tell me, let me know you were upset?" Mae Daeng told me to talk to Goy. I went to Goy's shop, and she reiterated what Mae Daeng had said and didn't elaborate. I was upset, but that afternoon, with Gaew and Sen's help, I found an old wooden house that one of Gaew's friends was renting in a village on the other end of town where Mae Daeng's twin lived, a friend of a friend's place, and started to move in. After I had spent just one night at the new house, though, Mae Daeng came to see me. "I had a dream," she said. "I dreamt something happened to you. I dreamt I was a bad mom. You should come back and live with me again."

"But what about the things I did wrong?" I asked, "I need to know ahead of time about them. I'll try to change, to be a better person. Tell me when something is wrong ahead of time—it's the way I'm used to things at home, OK?"

She nodded vaguely. "Don't worry about it," she replied. I went to talk to Goy. "*Jai yen*," she said. "Don't stress about it," she went on, laughing. "You think too much!"

I was confused: either I should worry about the situation, think and try to change the way I had been acting, or not worry about it and continue on as before. I spent a long afternoon talking with Sen, who was minding the family shop the whole afternoon while Gaew and their parents were stocking supplies in Chiang Mai. "Don't think about it, don't talk about it," he said, as I sat at the desk thinking and talking about it, pausing only when customers came in to buy something. "Don't keep it inside," he said. "*Jai yen*." It seemed like a contradiction: first I was told not to let it out, and then I was told not to keep it in. But later I came to realize that the point was not about an inside and an outside and where to "keep" a feeling; the goal was to not keep it at all.

I moved back into Mae Daeng's house and tried to come home earlier and do things more "correctly." After that experience I started paying more attention to my own emotions along with others', noting how people reacted to them. I was used to feeling an emotion and then either keeping it in or letting it out, according to my own cultural theory about how the mind works, but in Mae Jaeng, at least for Mae Daeng and Goy, a different kind of process seemed to be involved. While trying to orient myself to this new place, I had occasionally expressed my discontent, as when the food I ordered at a food stall wasn't ready because the person making it kept having friends show up to chat, or when the internet shop lost the work I had done because of an error they had promised to correct. In these instances I had said exactly what I felt: I spoke directly, in a strong tone, voicing my complaint to exert my will and get what I felt was my due. Even from early on in my stay, however, I felt that there was something off about these performances: the way people looked at me and each other, with slightly disdainful, bemused expressions. I was made to feel wrong to engage in them. One night as we were having dinner, Gaew's aunt asked me to teach her son English, and as it seemed to be the millionth time plus one that this request had been made by the people around me, I said, exasperated, "No! I'm not here as an English teacher!"

Gaew's aunt smiled tensely and became quiet. Gaew pulled me aside afterward and reprimanded me: "You shouldn't have said that, Julia. You should smile, agree, and be done with it." The important part was the affect, not the behavior. It was almost irrelevant if I actually followed through on the arrangement I was supposed to agree to. Over time, instances like this of doing emotion "wrong" taught me almost unconsciously to stop my emotional displays: I learned to laugh even when I said something serious; I learned to smile when I felt something sad.

Soon, however, it was not just displays that I was changing. Soon I didn't just put on a "face," but actually felt these things. I learned not to say something serious, or even to feel serious about it in the first place. I learned not to be sad even when I sometimes felt the situation called for it. Months after Mae Daeng had almost kicked me out of the house, I was talking to Sen, who told me he had just overheard Mae Daeng telling his mother that I had gotten better.

"Better?" I asked, taken aback. "Better how?" I was surprised that I wasn't "good" to begin with.

"Well . . . she said you're more Thai now." When I pushed for further elaboration, curious about what her image of "Thai-ness" might be, he said, "You're more *jai yen*." It turned out that Mae Daeng was talking about precisely this aspect of emotion, of calmness and a "cool heart."

Right around the time that instances of calmness were fading into the taken-for-granted everydayness of culture and failing to strike my attention, a visit from Laina, the twenty-year-old niece of an American friend, cast the concept into relief. My American friend had e-mailed, asking if I could host his niece for a few days, and a week later she showed up, eager to experience "traditional" Thailand. After a day of learning to drive my motorbike while I was off interviewing (with adventures on dirt paths of various hillside monasteries and a close call with a ditch by a rice field), Gaew, Gaew's friend Aung, Laina, and I went to P'Na's place for dinner, one of Mae Jaeng's two restaurants. Over barbecued pork and vegetables by the river, the four of us talked about Thailand, politics, and Buddhism. Gaew and Aung practiced what English they knew, and Laina told us about her travel plans for the coming month. "I'm going to go traveling around the north here. I'll just stay overnight in monasteries I find on the way," Laina said. I was a little bit skeptical of her plan, and I told her so.

"You can't do that," I said. "You can't just show up at a wat somewhere and expect them to host you, especially you as a woman!" I had seen so many international visitors to Thailand act in ways that were contrary to what I perceived to be proper for Thai Buddhist culture, and I wanted to protect the local norms from someone who would not know the correct etiquette but would probably be humored by the kindness of hosts anyway.

"Yeah, well I researched it online before coming here," she retorted. "You shouldn't act like you know everything about Northern Thailand!" The discussion became heated, but it was compelling, and interesting. We talked animatedly about propriety and knowledge, and perceptions about states of religious practice, about what was right and wrong and expected, and how one could find these things out. It reminded me of discussions I had back home in my graduate program at the University of Chicago, about ideas and opinions and perspectives that were at odds with one another. The dialogue was refreshing, even if it was intense.

After dinner, as the four of us were walking home, Gaew and Aung sidled up to me, a little wide-eyed, and Gaew whispered: "You guys were fighting! Is everything OK between the two of you?" I was surprised, and told Laina what Gaew had said.

Laina and I laughed and put our arms around each other's shoulders to show Gaew and Aung camaraderie. "We're fine," I told them. "We were just talking; we're friends."

Gaew and Aung nodded, a bit perplexed. Their worried reaction made me realize the absence of heated, intense discussions among my friends and informants in Mae Jaeng. Gaew, Aung, Sen, and Goy of course all had differing opinions about things, but there wasn't the same desire to talk it out or discuss or persuade as I was used to. Ta's presence in our house called attention to common practices by disrupting them. My animated disagreement with Laina did the same.

In our own ways Ta, Laina, and I were all oddities in Mae Jaeng. Ta was odd for his mental idiosyncrasies and past drug use, and Laina and I were odd for our foreignness (and for idiosyncrasies of our own). I wanted to find others who didn't quite fit in, to see through the foil of their actions and others' responses to them.

I thought that children would be an obvious site to find instances where emotions were expressed impulsively. Children, I thought, would be taught by others, through the process of acculturation, to act more "calmly" than they would normally. Developmental psychologists attend to the practices surrounding the enculturation of children as they are trained to become socially fluent adults. Children, I figured, could be seen as the most in need of explicit cultural instruction to cover up emotion. Although children weren't seen to automatically have more hot or impatient emotions than adults, there was a tendency in interviews to connect hot-heartedness to a kind of immaturity, and cool-heartedness to a mature person:

> When [my brother] was young he had a *jai ron*, a hot *arom* [mood]. . . . He's better now though, he's *jai yen* more. Because he's an adult, because he has a family; he can't make his wife mad or upset.

> My *arom* was hot-hearted when I was a teenager. If I wanted to do something, I had to finish it, I had to do it. I would do things fast and finish them fast. But I'm older now, and it's better.

It seemed that a "mature" person was cool-hearted. But when I asked Gaew about how parents train their children away from loudness and robust emotions, she looked at me, amused, and corrected my presumption of a more hot-hearted person hiding under, or previous to, the encultur-ated person. She said, laughing almost derisively, "Why do you think they would be loud like American children? Americans raise their kids to be loud, but not us; we're just regular and natural." I had fallen into the trap of thinking my way was natural and normal, as we may all be prone to do, and that it was others who were in need of explanations for variances from it; and Gaew was doing the same thing.

When I looked at the children around me, even the ones I knew well seemed relatively quiet, more so than the children I knew back home who ran around, screamed, cried, demanded, and generally "emoted" with vigor. One week about six months into my stay, Mae Daeng's niece Niw came to visit from New Jersey, where she had been living since graduating from college in Bangkok a few years earlier. She brought her two-year-old son Kuni, who wreaked cute havoc, talking loudly, demanding his mother pick him up, and playing exuberantly with his cousins. When I asked Kuni's doting grandmother Mae Lah, Mae Daeng's sister, how the visit was going, she said, half smiling as she laid out a cultural stereotype, "He's a bit too . . . American."

The crafting of a cool heart may be a particularly Buddhist practice, but because in everyday life in Mae Jaeng people did not tend to include the abstract terms of textual Pali Buddhist teachings outside of formal religious settings, I couldn't be confident that my conclusions connecting the two were more than a general feeling. I wanted to compare the emotions around me with a group of people who were similar but did things differently.[1] I needed a comparison group, and children weren't it.

"Why don't you go to Ban Ko Tao?" Gaew suggested when I explained the problem to her. "It's a Karen village, and Christian. My dad used to teach there when he worked as a teacher for the government. They're nice." Because Ban Ko Tao was Karen it would have a different ethnic and cultural background and wouldn't be a "perfect" comparison group;

---

1. Americans (usually American college students) typically serve as the comparative group for U.S.-based cross-cultural research in the psychological sciences, and I considered making an American group my comparison case, but there seemed to be so many variables at play that isolating religion as a relevant one would in the end just be speculation. I wanted something closer to Mae Jaeng. I had thought about doing research in a Muslim village called Mae Salong about three hours north of Mae Jaeng, but I had been advised that the time away from fieldwork in Mae Jaeng would make the main focus of study weaker. I had spoken with Christian groups in the city of Chiang Mai, but their scattered households seemed too integrated within the larger Buddhist majority of the city, and were so much more tied to urban lifestyles, that it seemed it would be difficult to gauge religious connections in affect among them.

but in many senses, including livelihood, environment, and nationality, it was very similar to Mae Jaeng without following Buddhism. I decided to check it out.

Talking, Singing, and the Culturally Variable Art of Not Burning in Hell: Emotion in a Karen, Christian Village

"You'll have to bring some food with you," Mae Daeng said when I told her I was about to travel the ten kilometers between Mae Jaeng town and Ban Ko Tao. "They don't have anything to eat up there." I looked at her, about to laugh, but she seemed serious. With a packed lunch of sticky rice and vegetables, I headed out to Mae Ko Tah on my motorcycle, turning off the main road a few kilometers on, at a corner marked by a sparkling wat and a spirit shrine by a waterfall, then snaking past the Buddhist neighborhood of Ban Toh Rua and driving up a long dirt road to the fifty households or so that make up the Karen village. A woman was minding a shop at the place where the dirt road forked and a cluster of houses stood out from the woods.

"*Sawatdii*"—"Hello!" a woman with long, swinging black hair called out in Thai, and I went over to talk with her. She shook my hand and smiled and said hello again, this time in Karen: "*Tablu!*" Her name was Duansri. She was my age, with two daughters—an eight-year-old, Min, who was funny and gregarious, and twelve-year-old May, who was shy and sweet. That day, like most others, Duansri was dressed in work boots and a plaid shirt and jeans, having just come back from harvesting in the *rai* hillside rice fields that were a little different from the lowland fields in Mae Jaeng but that still did, contrary to Mae Daeng's opinion, produce delicious food. It was a weekday that first day, but on Sundays Duansri and everyone else would dress up in traditional V-neck Karen outfits of woven cloth and go to church. Like Mae Daeng, Duansri had a lot of brothers and sisters, fifteen in all, all of them still living in the village. In addition to working in the fields, she also wove cloth, shucked fruits, gathered mushrooms in the woods, and sold goods at the shop, basically doing whatever was useful to the family.

When foreigners arrive to visit in Ban Ko Tao, I learned, they usually stay at the home of Duansri's cousin Jerapong, the pastor of the wooden church at the top of the hill. But Duansri and I took a liking to each other right away, and by the second visit she had opened her home to me. "You can stay here at our house whenever you're in Ban Ko Tao."

The first Christian in the village was Duansri's grandfather. His grave is in the cemetery in the woods at the edge of the village, and is regularly visited by his many children and many more grandchildren and great-grandchildren. As a community of people only ten kilometers from Mae Jaeng with a non-Buddhist religious tradition, Ban Ko Tao seemed like a good place to look at non-Buddhist ideas in practice.[2]

Every Wednesday evening and twice on Sunday Jerapong led services at the Christian Baptist church overlooking the village. Jerapong's uncle was an old man named Paw Pu, who had been the previous pastor and the father of Duansri and her siblings. Pu was the patriarch of the village and the son of the village's first Christian convert, and while he was friendly he was also in his eighties and slowing down; Jerapong was the charismatic de facto leader of the village. Jerapong was often invited to represent the "poor hill tribe of Thailand" in the host countries of the missionaries that regularly passed through, and unlike anyone else I knew in the area— few of whom had made it as far as Bangkok—he had already visited the United States, Jerusalem, England, and Australia.

Duansri and her daughters brought me to church on Sundays dressed in the white robes called *che gua* that unmarried girls wore. At the church, the service began with a song from the children's choir, and for the next hour Jerapong offered readings and explanations from the Bible interspersed with choirs and music from a full band of drums and guitars played by the parishioners. Duansri and I sat together every week and whispered to each other and the neighbors, picking up toddlers who had wandered

---

2. Population estimate accessed from http://www.peoplegroups.org/Explore/groupdetails. aspx?peid=10917 on September 5, 2014. These numbers vary widely, however, and should be seen more as an approximation than an exact count. Census-taking practices, ethnic identifications, and movements between and within Thai and Burmese communities make exact counts difficult. For more information on Christian Karen practices in Northern Thailand see Hayami 2004, Platz 2003, Hovemyr 1989, Loo Shwe 1962, and broader analyses of Christian and Karen history. Khwanchewan Buandaeng's *Buddhism, Christianity, and the Ancestors: Religion and Pragmatism in a Skaw Karen Community of North Thailand* (2003) offers ethnographic descriptions of the village described here, and my research assistant's book *Ruanglaojakphucow* (Stories told from the hills) (Chuchuhnjitsakun 2004) offers descriptions of cultural practices and a history of Karen in the region.

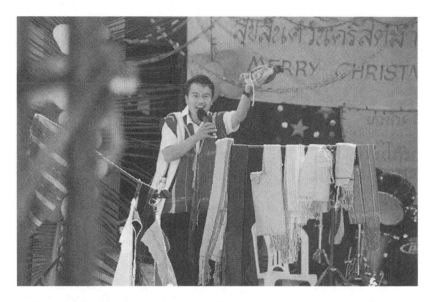

Figure 7. The Christian community in Ban Ko Tao gathers for a Christmas celebration;
here the pastor auctions a chicken to raise money for the church.

over and sometimes opening up a Bible to follow along with the music
and words. After church, people mingled around the top of the hill, where
it was slightly cooler than down below, and food was made for lunch. A
second, Catholic church nearby was attended by approximately 25 percent
of the people in the village. When I asked Jerapong if there were any tensions between the Protestant majority and the Catholic minority, he said
"sometimes there are a few issues, but those are problems with people, not
with God."

One morning during a Sunday church service Jerapong announced that
a Baptist Christian missionary from Kansas was in town and would be saying a few words to the congregation. Missionaries from places like America, Australia, or Korea are fairly common in Ban Ko Tao, unlike in Mae
Jaeng, where foreigners passing through are rare (and cause talk and even
suggestions by Gaew or Aung that we invite them out to dinner). Foreigners in Ban Ko Tao arrived almost monthly to stay at Jerapong's house and
support the villagers by preaching the gospel and donating money.

The woman from Kansas stood up at the podium that morning and
started to speak enthusiastically. She didn't know Karen or Thai, so she

spoke in English, and Jerapong, who was the only person in Ban Ko Tao other than me who understood English, translated her words directly into Karen for the listening congregation. The woman became more and more riled as she spoke, her face turning red from the heat and her animated speech. She waved her hands in the air and told us about fire and brimstone and an angry God and the importance of following his word. I felt uncomfortable with the energy of her discourse, being more used to the relatively calmer tone around me during typical Sunday services. At one point she started talking about the people in Ban Toh Rua, the Buddhist Northern Thai village a few kilometers down the hill from Ban Ko Tao on the way to Mae Jaeng.

"We have to convert those people down there to Christianity!" the missionary said, "or else they'll all burn in Hell!"

I was taken aback by her tone, and curious what the others were thinking about what she was saying. My Karen language skills weren't good enough at that point to follow Jerapong's translation directly, but the message in English was clear to me. I leaned over to Duansri, who was sitting next to me playing with the hair of a toddler in the chair in front of us, and asked her in Thai what she thought.

"Oh, she's funny," Duansri said. "It's entertaining to see new things around here." This was the kind of response I heard regularly when people spoke of the strange behaviors of Thailand's international visitors, as amusing oddities to be humored, but I had thought that this time the missionary's message would have evoked a stronger reaction. Duansri went back to her hair braiding, half listening as the woman wound up her speech.

After the church service I approached Jerapong and asked what he thought of the missionary's comments. He gave me a similar response.

"But what about what she said about the people in Ban Toh Rua?" I pushed, "That if they're not Christian they'll burn in hell? How did you feel about translating that?" It was such a striking sentiment, and it seemed to go against the more tolerant tenor of religion I felt in the valley.

Jerapong looked at me and said, "Oh, I didn't translate *that* part!"

I was surprised, and he went on, "I mean, those are our friends down the road. All religion teaches one to be a good person. I didn't want people to get upset or anything or think otherwise." I laughed, a little bit taken aback, and he looked at me and smiled. I went back to find Duansri and make lunch, and spent the rest of the afternoon at her shop thinking about what he had said.

Jerapong's comment was telling of so much that was going on around me. It pointed to the blending and blurring of influences in the two communities of Ban Ko Tao and Mae Jaeng. The Christian community was not isolated from the Buddhist one—even with the relatively more robust emotional tone in Ban Ko Tao, the two villages were influenced by common histories. I had heard the phrase "all religion teaches one to be a good person" often in Mae Jaeng and Ban Ko Tao, and after I mentioned to Goy how frequently I heard it she told me that it was something that everyone learned in school. I later found the exact phrase in one of the textbooks used in the national school curriculum that Karen and Northern Thai children both learned from: "Every religion teaches one to be a good person."

Jerapong's comment made me realize that the imagined Christian community, even in the same denomination, was not of a single nature, nor understood to exist more authoritatively in a foreign land or a foreign country. Just because an American missionary said that Christianity meant one thing, his comment seemed to imply, it wasn't necessarily the case that it was true for Christianity in Ban Ko Tao. Jerapong's comment pointed out that even though multiple voices can be thought of as true, knowledge and ideas still always sift through structures of power and privilege. It was Jerapong's choice as the powerful pastor to choose what to relay or not relay. Duansri had told me that her father, the old pastor Paw Pu, felt a little disenfranchised with his inability to speak Thai and take part in the increasingly global community of the church that Jerapong was becoming more and more conversant in. Jerapong made a choice about what to present in the service; and I from knowing him was privileged to hear his reasoning. The people in the position to speak are the people whose perspectives are heard.

Sometimes in the evenings when May, Min, and I left Duansri's with a flashlight to get something at Jerapong's house, or just to say hello to him and his wife Sada, we would all sit for a while in their living room and look through pictures from Jerapon's trips abroad or listen to someone in his family playing guitar, or talk about problems he and his family were going through. The exchange about the visiting missionary reminded me how worthwhile it was to spend a significant amount of time in Ban Ko Tao and get to know the people in it. Had I just visited and taken interviews and left, Jerapong never would have gotten comfortable enough with me to tell me he intentionally mistranslated a guest's words. And I liked spending time with Jerapong and Sada; it was comfortable and felt free.

On my weekend visits to Ban Ko Tao I stayed at Duansri's house and spent time at her shop at the main intersection, as I did with Gaew and Sen. Breaking with tradition and the wishes of her father, Duansri had married a Northern Thai man, P'Duang, who like most Northern Thai men had moved into his wife's household, and now bought and sold buffalo for work, heading off to the remote hills in the mornings with an animal or two in the back of his truck. P'Duang was the only Buddhist and the only Northern Thai person living in the village; everyone else was S'gaw Karen, the most populous branch of the Karen ethnic group in Thailand, and most were Baptist Christian. At night P'Duang, May, and Min practiced English with me when I was staying over, laughing at the seeming impossibility of mastering the sounds of the language, or we watched TV and talked. Sometimes at night the kids went to their grandfather's house for church music practice with groups of others, and the sounds of the singing and guitar could be heard throughout the village.

Unlike my host family and friends in Mae Jaeng, who referred to where I came from vaguely as *muang nok*, "the land outside," and who rarely if ever asked about what life was like there, Duansri, P'Duang, and others I was getting to know in Ban Ko Tao asked regularly about what snow felt like, and what my government was up to, and what it was like to travel back and forth to America. "If I'm in California," Sada asked me one day as she was preparing a visa application to travel to the United States, "let's say I wanted to fly from California to Los Angeles—how long would that take?" I started to laugh, but then I realized how little I knew about regions of the world I had never been to either.

On Sundays after church Duansri and her family stayed around the shop house shucking fruits and vegetables and chatting as people passed by. Sometimes they hiked in the woods or swam at the bottom of waterfalls, and always shared eagerly in gossip. Like in Mae Jaeng, shops served as ideal locations to watch people go about their daily business. Virtually everyone in town stopped by during the day, as the shop was the only store around and was the last building before the dirt path led out of the village. Passersby usually stayed to chat with each other, chew the ubiquitous legal narcotic of the betel-nut leaf, wait for a neighbor to bring them into town, take a phone call on the village's one telephone, or lie down to rest from the hot sun. During the weekdays the children went to school and adults went to work in their rice fields scattered around the hillside, but Sunday was always a day of rest.

I could easily sense a different emotional tenor in Ban Ko Tao from that in Mae Jaeng. Like the wats of Mae Jaeng, the church in Ban Ko Tao is the social center for the community; even P'Duang, Duansri's husband and the only non-Karen, non-Christian man in the village, would sometimes take part in church-sponsored events, including clearing the brush around the hilltop to make room for a soccer field, or participating in the church's "sport day." But unlike the quiet that was cultivated in the Buddhist wats, emotional energy filled the Christian churches in Ban Ko Tao.

Jerapong's church sermons were full of feeling, effervescent even, as were the music and the participation of the congregation, some of whom played the drums, guitar, and other instruments onstage and almost half of whom came up to the front of the church to sing at some point during the service, often speaking up with thoughts or prayers, talking about their personal struggles and ideas.

Even with the reminder about the culturally embedded, Thai-influenced nature of religious practice in Ban Ko Tao that Jerapong had offered through the missionary, I still felt a different, more heated emotional tone. People talked more about feelings, their faces were more animated, and they spoke directly to each other about their emotions. A visiting American Peace Corps worker I came across in Mae Jaeng noticed this too; when I asked her about her impression of the people in the area she said that while both the Buddhists and the Christians seemed equally "into" their religion, the Christians seemed more "enthusiastic."[3]

---

3. "Enthusiasm" has a colloquial English meaning today but ties in to some forms of Christian religious experience. From the Greek *en-thous*, enthusiasm originally referred to the experiences of people who believed themselves to be possessed by a god, but its meaning gradually expanded, and by the tenth to seventeenth centuries the word came to be defined by not just god possession but also as intense religious fervor and emotion. Ann Taves writes of the French prophets in England in the 1700s in the enthusiastic religious tradition characterized by bodily agitations (Taves 2011). In the seventeenth and eighteenth centuries many Protestants began to emphasize direct religious experience and as such were accused of being enthusiasts; they both distanced themselves from such accusations and were influenced by enthusiastic perspectives. In her use of the term, the Peace Corps volunteer I spoke with referred less to these overt Christian references and more to a sense of robust emotionality in the Karen communities, full of loud church music and animated discussion, as compared with the Buddhist Thai communities, with the sense of quiet that pervades monastery spaces.

TABLE 2. Interview demographics in the Karen Christian communities

	Ban Ko Tao	Mae Ma Law
Religion	Christian	Christian
Setting	Village near town	Very rural
Number of people interviewed	30	30
Average age	42	38
Male / female	M 14 / F 16	M 16 / F 14
Average schooling	9th grade high school	5th grade elementary

I decided to extend my interviews to include Ban Ko Tao. Like in Mae Jaeng, the interviews would provide a broader range of input than would be possible from conversations with a small group of friends and general observations of others. Ari and I found a Karen man named Chalong fifty kilometers away who had crossed the border from Burma; he was proficient in typing the Karen script on a computer keyboard, and we worked with him to translate and type up the Thai and English interview into the Karen S'gaw language that the older people in the village read, substituting "church" for "wat" in the religion questions. We started to visit Ban Ko Tao together and interview those willing to speak with us, which turned out to be virtually everyone we came across. About 80 percent of the people interviewed knew Thai, but we asked them to speak during the interview in whatever language they felt more comfortable with, as Ari knew Karen and could help translate. We decided to also interview people in Mae Ma Law, a village thirty kilometers farther up in the mountains, past Mae Wak, that had no electricity or paved roads, to get a better sense of the diversity within the Karen communities in the area.

As expected, people in the Karen communities talked about the calmness of a cool heart, but they also and much more than in the Buddhist interviews in Mae Jaeng discussed expressive, robust, even sometimes "hot" emotions. Often emotion in the Karen communities was framed in terms of speaking or expressing feelings, and even the value of doing so:

My brother helps out with raising the buffalo. He has a good personality, he speaks a lot.

When I was young I didn't speak much, but when I was older I would talk more. I was brave enough to speak, and talk about things that people would say that weren't right.

My brother talks a lot, he sees a lot, he has a big personality. People come to him with their problems.

This emotional orientation was also common when people talked about their reasons for attending church:

I go to church because I have happiness when I go to church; I thank God, I ask God to help.

A friend in Mae Jaeng had said in passing, "Those people in Ban Ko Tao, they talk a lot about themselves; they're so self-centered." People in Ban Ko Tao in turn made a similar moral comment about opposite emotional practices: "Mae Jaeng people don't do much hard work, they're so lazy, all *jai yen*." The sentiments of emotion and their values were clearly marked in the two communities, and the relatively more robust emotional tone, even heat, in Ban Ko Tao made the cool-heartedness in Mae Jaeng even more apparent. A *jai yen* wasn't just a national project or a universally human practice; it was a religious and cultural one.

The Idiom of Heat and the Psychology of Emotion in Culture

One early morning in the cold season while it was still dark out, Goy, Mae Daeng, and I climbed into the back of a pickup truck and took off with a few neighbors to Ban Tap monastery on the edge of town for Wan Pow Lua Pa Jow, a traditional Northern Thai event that takes place every year at the height of the cold season. The drive to the temple was dark, with cool, quiet air whipping around us; we smiled in the dark and hid our faces from the wind. At the monastery, we found a bonfire burning about ten feet tall in the field. The group of us sat around the fire with about a hundred others, warming our hands as the sun slowly thought about rising, revealing through the mist the wat roof and the Buddha statue inside. As the monks chanted, I started chatting with an old woman wearing a bright green Chang Beer blanket over her shoulders. "Do you know why the monastery has this festival with the fire today?" she asked, curious if I knew the answer.
"Because it's a full moon today?" I guessed.

"It's a full moon every month. Why this month?"

"Because it's the fourth month [in the lunar calendar]?"

"Yeah, but why?" She didn't wait for my response this time. "It's because it's cold. It's the cold season."

"Oh," I said, not fully understanding.

She continued, "The Buddha at this time, you know the Buddha [Phra Phuttha Chao] is the Buddha image [Phra Phuttha Rup]. And the Buddha is cold."

"So they have a big bonfire to keep him warm?"

She smiled. "Yeah."

It was a pleasant image, the Buddha statue in the monastery becoming warmed by the fire in the field that predawn morning. The woman went on, "It's like when I go to the monastery, I go to warm my heart. Like this blanket: we have to put the blanket on ourselves; no one else will do it for us."

The woman's comment struck a chord with me. I had interviewed over fifty people by then, and almost all, when asked why they went to the monastery, mentioned something along the lines of "to cool my heart." This woman's sentiment described not coolness but warmth. Was she advocating a "hot heart," a *jai ron*? It didn't seem like it: she didn't seem excited, angry, or "impatient." Like the others, she seemed to be advocating a sense of calmness. I realized that the coolness of a *jai yen* is not coldness as Americans would mean by the term—describing, as it does in English, a kind of unfeeling distance and disdain. It was rather something more like a softening of sentiments, a move toward equilibrium. Using the metaphor of heat in this way suggested that extreme "coldness" and "heat" are equally and actively undesirable. The woman was talking initially about the physical discomfort of heat and cold, but what she meant was a mental orientation to emotion. While people in Mae Jaeng said they went to the monastery in order "to cool my heart" (or some variation thereof), in the cold dark morning at Wat Ban Tap the practice of going to the monastery instead is warming. It brings one in the opposite direction, away from whatever the nearest extreme might be, toward what Buddhist texts describe as "equanimity."

The warming of the Buddha image helped me to understand Goy's "cool" reaction to Ta dropping the furniture, and Mae Daeng's reaction to his stomping around the house. It is impossible to truly get into someone else's head, and I couldn't tell exactly what they were thinking and feeling, but from asking them and from knowing them as I did, I felt confident that they were not "angry" per se, or even "annoyed" exactly. It was not that Goy and her mother were "pushing down" anger or annoyance, keeping them inside. Something else was going on, a kind of affective drive like the attention to the warmth of the Buddha on a cold day. It was a coolness aimed less toward automatic or unfeeling cold, and more toward crafting a calm affective equilibrium.

I wanted to know about the psychology of emotion in Mae Jaeng, and the heat of hearts certainly seemed central; but was a "cool heart" or a "hot heart" even an emotion? It seemed more like a feeling that people had than a fully formed affective state. The Oxford dictionary had said that emotion is about riled agitation, but there is no similar definition in Thai. Thai-English dictionaries most often translate "emotion" as *khuam ruu suk* (feeling), or *arom* (mood), but neither quite captures the particular conjunction of ideas that go into the meaning of the English word. In hearing people talk about *anicca* as a guide for emotion, I had become intrigued about emotional life in Mae Jaeng, and I had anticipated that I could study it. But finding a Thai word for emotion turned out to be a much bigger task than I first anticipated. No one in Mae Jaeng speaks English, so the people I was living among couldn't help with the task. When I asked English speakers elsewhere in Thailand, they gave me the English-language term, complete with its implicit cultural meanings, and halfheartedly suggested some Thai words that "kind of" referred to emotion. The problem was not "simply" a problem of translation.

I went to talk with Ajarn Somwang, my friend and professor of philosophy and religion at Chiang Mai University, and asked him about emotion. He confirmed what I had already guessed: that there is no word for emotion in Thai at all.

"Emotion," Somwang told me, scoffing at the term and speaking in English when I asked him about it, "emotion is just a piece of psychological academic vocabulary; it doesn't mean anything here!" He pointed to the Psychology Department down the hall: "It's just a word they use." I had at that time an office in the Psychology Department to use when I was in town, just down the hall from Somwang's office, and I, like Somwang, was familiar with the kind of work going on there. They mostly re-created European and American psychology studies, ignoring or flattening out cultural difference. The head of the department was interested in the work I was doing but was hesitant to pursue similar research, perhaps because it wasn't seen to be as publishable as research that reproduced variations of established measures and results from the United States. By "psychological academic vocabulary," Ajarn Somwang was using "emotion" as a code word for an English-language-biased, U.S. psychology of emotion.

Without a comparable term in Thai it seemed that a study of emotion would be futile. But it did seem that people I encountered had feelings; they thought and felt in ways that at least seemed relatable. I asked Somwang to try to translate "emotion" into Thai, even though I couldn't find a suitable term in any dictionary, and he told me one didn't exist. "Emotion in Thai is . . . umm . . . *khuam ruu suk* [feeling], or *arom* [mood] . . . I guess," he said, citing terms that Thai-English dictionaries and other bilingual friends had also suggested. He tried elaborating: "We can think of emotion as involving a mix of sensation, feeling, and perception. It comes from *kam* [karma], from intention."

Not only is a clear translation of the word "emotion" absent in Thai; it is also absent in the Pali language of Buddhism. I recalled a Buddhist Thai friend and a Muslim Thai friend talking about religion once in Bangkok: the Muslim friend had explained a bit about his religion and Allah, and the Buddhist friend said in reply, "Well, we don't have anything that looks like that, but what we have is a way to do emotion." Emotional practice, he implied, *is* what Buddhism is about. In looking over Pali chanting books and English- and Thai-language translations of *suttas* (sutras, or discourses of the Buddha), commentaries, and analyses about thoughts and feelings, I thought, based on that conversation and others, that I would come across a lot of discussion, or at least a term that means "emotion." But there isn't one, and scholars of Buddhist texts agree: "There is no Sanskrit or Pali word that corresponds directly to the modern American idea of 'emotion'" (Rotman 2003, 556). In everyday conversations people in Mae Jaeng labeled certain perspectives on feeling as more or less Buddhist, but there is little textually to think of as officially "Buddhist" at the level of discrete states of experience. Unlike with impermanence, there is not an "official" or "doctrinal" discussion of emotions to use as a guide for understanding how people interact with official teachings.

If emotion is supposedly so basic, so universal, shouldn't there be a term for it in every language? That there is no clear, direct translation of "emotion" in Thai in itself suggests that what makes up emotion in English is not experienced the same way across cultures. This non-translatability is often ignored by cross-cultural psychologists and some anthropologists who may assume the epistemological status of an experiential state without asking whether it exists as a bound phenomenon in the same way in different cultural contexts. This oversight is a side effect, perhaps, of most psychologists working with just one language, usually English.

Psychologists who study emotion often talk about it as a process of internal, physiological experience that may then be "regulated" personally using cultural norms (Gross 1998; Carstensen, Isaacowitz, and Charles 1999; Ekman et al. 1987; Campos, Campos, and Barrett 1989). Anthropologists, when they talk about emotion at all, often talk about it as constructed by cultural discourses that happen outside, in the space of ideas, that are brought into bodies and minds.[4] These are two sides of the same coin, with one side emphasizing internal experience and the other emphasizing external social construction, but the two sides rarely meet in theoretical analyses. A good deal of work has been done by both psychologists and anthropologists to isolate basic, universal emotions, and at first in Mae Jaeng I had been seeking out evidence of the kinds of feelings I was used to: anger, sadness, happiness, or some of the other basic emotions that have been suggested, to then see how they were dealt with. But I was unable to make sense of emotionality in the community using these words and the accompanying idea that the emotions first happened and then were dealt with either through expression or suppression. Thai terms that could be mapped onto them, like *grot* for anger, *sao* for sadness, or *khwam suk* for happiness, were easy to find, and I could label experiences as reflecting

---

4. For more on social constructivist anthropological theories of emotion see Lutz 1988 and Lutz and White 1986. One difficulty with simply acknowledging cultural variation in talk about emotion is that this perspective fails to encapsulate the range of "emotion work" (Hochschild 1979) that goes on in different cultural contexts. But the idea of emotion work, even as it reveals an important side of social life, is itself problematic: like in Goffman's "presentation of self" (1959), the evidence behind the idea of emotion *work* is based on just that—the situation that arises when particular emotional countenances are part of one's (usually paid) labor, as both Goffman's and Hochschild's informants were. Analogies can be made to the work of culture in other contexts, but they are incomplete. Using them whole risks slipping back into the deterministic model of "culture masks over inner turmoil" (e.g., Obeyesekere 1990), returning to a universalizing, hydraulic model of emotion that suggests that people in some historical contexts are taught to fight the natural expression of their emotions.

them when I tried, but I found that this missed what was really happening in the emotional lives of people I knew.[5]

Scholars who have understood that the idea of basic universal emotions is problematic have instead suggested culturally specific focal emotions, as emotions that are especially elaborated in one cultural context, such as an avoidance of anger for Inuits (Briggs 1970), the rage in grief for Ifaluk (Rosaldo 1984), or the power of shame for Oriyas (Shweder 2003a). I wanted to find a similar "key emotion" in Mae Jaeng. At first I thought that the calmness of a "cool heart" was it. A cool heart is certainly marked and elaborated and more extensive in Mae Jaeng than elsewhere. But as pervasive as it was, it didn't feel quite like an emotion. It felt more like a process, or a part of emotion rather than a static, locally valued state.

Rather than as discrete emotions, experiences involving the heat of the heart in Mae Jaeng can be better understood through theoretical perspectives of the mind that take into account qualities of affect interpersonally shared in culture. There are many of these kinds of theories: cultural schema theory draws attention to scripts that incorporate values, attitudes, and social histories (Strauss and Quinn 1997); componential theories take into account aspects of feeling, including cognitive appraisals, interpersonal relations, and communication strategies in emotional experience (Shweder et al. 2008; Shweder 1994; Luhrmann 2006; Frijda 1988); affect theory shows how interpersonal energy is intersubjectively captured in the pushes and pulls of actions and reactions (Gregg and Seigworth 2010; Massumi 1995); and affective circumplex models take into account the moralized weight that valence and arousal carry as dimensions of feeling in cultural context (Russell 1980; Russell and Barrett 1999; Posner, Russell, and Peterson 2005; Tsai 2007). They help to capture the interpersonal, moralized, and processional quality of emotionality in Mae

---

5. This is not unusual—even Ekman, often considered the founder of the idea of universal emotionality, in designing his forced-choice tasks that were bent on showing universal basic emotions (which he claims as anger, disgust, fear, shame, joy, sadness, and surprise), said that "it has not been easy to obtain adequate translations in every language even for the six or seven emotion words we have used in our studies" (Ekman 1994, 274). This alone suggests that emotions might not be universal, and, especially in a language that does not categorize affect in ways that quite map onto the English term, that they may not exist as discrete and static states at all (see also Wierzbicka 2013, 1999). Emotions may not be "basic," but rather are *always* culturally particular and contextual, having to do more with interpersonal relations than states.

Jaeng, highlighting the high value placed on low arousal in the idiom of the cool heart.[6]

Discussions of feelings in this sense are similarly everywhere in Buddhist teachings. The category of feelings, or *vedanā* in Pali, is one of five aggregates thought to make up a sense of self. In the Abhidhamma, the Tripitaka texts of Buddhist psychology, they are described as the affective quality of sensations and are characterized as pleasant, unpleasant, or neutral (Bhikkhu Bodhi 2003; De Silva [1979] 2000, 42).[7] It is through attachments to these *vedanā* as affective reactions to sensations that one develops what might in English be thought of as emotion—a felt attitude toward an object (a person, thing, event, or idea) involving bodily changes and particular tendencies to act in certain ways. The Abhidhamma suggests that feelings emerge from a relationship between senses and ideas, suggesting a construction rather than a reaction to events.[8]

---

6. Feelings of a cool heart are clearly idealized in Mae Jaeng (and "hypercognized" [Levy 1973]), yet one might think that they can be best understood simply as ideals that don't actually touch experience—cultural aspirations that only mask more universal internal psychological processes. But ideals are not abstract or intangible aspirations; the psychologists Batja Mesquita and Janxin Leu point to this when they remind us that emotions are not just experiences that "happen" to occur: "Cultural representations of emotions," they say, "especially focal emotions, emotion norms, and ideal affect, motivate the experience of emotions. They do so by facilitating positively valued emotional experiences and inhibiting negative emotional experiences" (2007, 753). Ideals can be understood to serve as guides, with social reinforcements and religious rituals serving as iterated and reiterated opportunities for practice. It is in this way that ideals become inscribed within experience. And it is the sense of emotional construction, of emotion making, rather than the separating of it from the actor and situation, that reveals the interaction of experience and ideas in particular circumstances. Such patterned and practiced emotion construction is part of the techniques of the self (Foucault 1980), and "structured, structuring dispositions" that Pierre Bourdieu calls the *habitus*, a system of shared, embodied habits that are less explicitly idealistic and more implicitly developed in the ways that people attend to their own and each other's feelings (1990, 52).

7. It is in this sense that the Buddhist Thai friend talking to the Muslim Thai friend in Bangkok meant that the cultivation of emotion is central to the Buddhist religion. David Webster writes in *The Philosophy of Desire in the Buddhist Pali Canon*, "Emotional responses are vitally important to Buddhism, so much so that we might argue that the Buddhist project is an attempt to train the emotions, rather than suppress or eliminate them" (2005, 119). For more on affective processes in textual Buddhist thought see Webster 2005, Kuan 2008, and De Silva 2000.

8. In a series of essays on emotion in Buddhism in the *Journal of the American Academy of Religion* (Gay 2003), a similar collective point is made that emotion as understood in Buddhists texts is constructivist and categorically different from the automatic agitations that English definitions of emotion usually invoke. Drawing on sources as far-ranging as the Divyāvadāna (a collection of Sanskrit Indian Buddhist narratives) and *vamsas* (Sri Lankan Buddhist histories), and the insights of Catherine Lutz, Martha Nussbaum, and other cultural theorists, the special issue argues

Cool hearts are valued in Mae Jaeng, but this does not mean that calmness reflects weak emotions (or "passive" emotions, as the stereotype may go), nor that emotion isn't felt as "strongly" in Mae Jaeng as elsewhere. Gaew corrected such an idea as we sat watching some European travelers talking loudly together on the street. "Why aren't people in Mae Jaeng as emotional as *farang?*" I asked, referring to the tourists with the Thai word for people of the "West."

"The reason Thai people don't seem as emotional is that Thai people feel stronger than *farang,*" she answered. Gaew's point is interesting for thinking about the strength of emotion; it is not "strong emotions" that people refrain from, she was suggesting, but the strength rather than weakness of low-arousal emotion that is practiced and aspired to in Mae Jaeng.

The same day Goy and Mae Daeng had asked me to leave their house, Sen's good friend Chai, who ran a freelance medical clinic in town, was sitting at the shop house with Sen watching the day pass by. Chai had noticed when he stopped by earlier that I was upset at something Goy had said, but now he turned to me and asked, "Gone yet?"

At first I wasn't sure what he meant. I asked him to clarify, and he said, "Are you still feeling bad, or is it gone yet?" *I'm still feeling bad—it's not gone*, I wanted to reply; *I haven't done anything with it yet!* I hadn't expressed the feeling of being upset, or figured out how to handle it, or understood what it meant, or anything. He was asking as if he felt that the feeling would just float away, or evaporate. People in Mae Jaeng do not think of controlling emotions by pushing them "down" or keeping them "inside." Instead they think of emotionality as diffuse and inchoate moods that can potentially overtake the body and mind for more or less intense

---

for a cultural psychological perspective on emotion in Buddhism, and that emotion is constructed through multiple components rather than instantaneously experienced. Similarly, in a commentary to a collection of articles titled "Passionate about Buddhism: Contesting Theories of Emotion," Volney Gay (2003) pits scholarly evolutionary determinism and postmodern constructivism at two ends of a spectrum and argues that Buddhist texts lend support to a moderate constructivist interpretation of emotion. In my own experience participating in a range of Buddhist practices, I have noticed that those following more northern forms of Buddhism (e.g., Tibetan or Zen) often think of emotions as more instantaneous and discrete than they are in Theravada thought: I am told that an emotion, practically fully formed, will arise, and the Buddhist practice regarding it is to keep from becoming attached to it by simply watching it arise and pass away rather than attach to it. In Theravada practices I hear this idea of fully formed emotions much less, and the idea of dealing with unformed feelings much more often.

(but always brief) periods before evaporating in the air.[9] This evaporation seems to happen to a feeling as it moves off from the skin of the mind and body; the metaphor suggests a boundary between the self and other, but a permeable one. The Thai phrase Chai used to ask the question, *hai ruu yang*, doesn't even have a subject—in the Thai there is not an *it* that is the subject or emotion that is then let go of. Instead of a discrete emotion like anger or worry, the phrase suggests something more like an amorphous feeling, or mood. Instead of explaining to him that I was upset I just grumbled. A few minutes later, though, I realized that the feeling, or mood, about the situation at Goy's house had in fact dissipated, and I felt cool and calm about it. Such an experience, I think, reflects the practice and process of emotionality in Mae Jaeng. But why, and how?

---

9. Clifford Geertz (1973b, 97) discusses moods in a similar sense: like fogs that settle, or like scents that diffuse and evaporate. This is not the "letting off steam" of yelling and expressing emotion, but a different kind of evaporation of vague moods moving away.

Part II

ATTACHMENT

3

LETTING GO

I was sitting in my room at Goy's house one afternoon, trying to angle the fan toward me and get at any breeze at all to help cool down in the stifling weather. The heat was oppressive, and I finally left the room to find Goy in the kitchen.

"It's too hot!" I complained.

"It's the hot season," she said. "It's hot out."

"But it's too hot!" I said, sitting down and looking at her desperately. "I don't know what to do! What should I do?" I was sweating; she seemed as calm and cool as ever. She barely seemed concerned. It was as if she didn't care. I was angry, too; angry at the heat, at her, at Mae Jaeng.

"Turn on a fan," she suggested, and I rolled my eyes at the idea that a fan hadn't already occurred to me. "You can't change the heat," Goy said, nonchalantly, before turning back to her bowl of food. "You have to let go, you have to *tham jai*."

I glared at her: how would *that* help! I got up and went back in my room, livid, to suffer in heat and anger. But the terms Goy used, to let go, and *tham jai* ("to make the heart"), stayed in my mind. "Making the heart" and letting go are part of affective orientations to everyday events and religious rituals alike. They are part of a complex of ideas revolving around the positive effects of acceptance, nonattachment, and an awareness of the inevitability of change.

Tham Jai: "Let Go and Make Your Heart"

The phrase "letting go" can be found in popular works on Buddhism in the United States and Thailand alike. A quick search at Amazon.com yields more than 36,608 hits for books containing the keywords "letting go"; more than a thousand of those books have these words in the title alone.[1] The positive implications surrounding the concept of letting go are fairly well known, but its meanings and the processes that are part of it are often left unelaborated, or given objective, acultural status. "Letting go" can be taken to mean, for instance, releasing of feelings by crying them out; dropping them to turn to something else; or distancing from someone whom you thought you knew, or from who you yourself had been. Letting go can be viewed in these popular renderings in different ways: as part of a languid, go-with-the-flow, mystical, New Age-y East; as a prescription self-help pill for mental health; as passive resignation from someone on the losing side of an argument; or as an ideal designed to control the masses as described by political scientists and religious skeptics. It is an ideal with a long history of analysis and aspiration in Buddhist texts, which speak of it in reference to nonattachment and the detriments of clinging (in Pali, *upadana*) to things that change. But while the usefulness of letting go is elaborated extensively in religious accounts, there is less to be found on how it works within the context of everyday life. I wanted less to learn about how it *should* work than how it *does* work for people in Mae Jaeng, because it seemed to connect an awareness of change to the calmness of a cool heart.

Ploy is a colloquial Thai, and not explicitly Buddhist, word that means "to let go." It is often paired with other words in a combined form, including *plod-ploy*, "to release, liberate." The most common combination I've

---

1. Data accessed online at amazon.com, January 12, 2014.

heard is *ploywang*, "to empty, to not take something to heart." *Plong*, to dispose of, to lay down a burden, is also used in reference to letting go. Both *ploy* and *plong* as colloquial references to letting go came up again and again in interviewee responses to questions about people and feelings.

> My brother used to like to lecture me when I was little, he used to tell me what to do. Now, though, through *ploy*-ing, he's let go.

> At sixty years old a person will know life, they'll have seen everything now, they can *plong*, they don't need to be as eager.

> [In the future] for me I'll *plong*, let go. Each day as it passes, I'll accept [*tham jai*].

When I first heard the term *plong* in an interview, and I asked Ari what it meant, he said simply, "*Plong* means . . . *tham jai*—to make the heart," the same thing that Goy had told me to do when I felt too hot in the house.

Goy told me to *tham jai* when she suggested turning on a fan; to let it go and accept the heat. Others talked about *tham jai* similarly, as a symbol or metaphor for accepting things that have happened. "Making the heart" is a way to talk about the emotional process of coming to terms with something, but is more than just a feeling; it is an orientation to feelings centered on the letting go of affective attachments. It is raised when people talk about how they have felt, and especially how they've dealt with loss.

One woman I knew had gone out into the woods searching for mushrooms, as so many people in her village do, and after weeks of foraging she brought them to the market to sell:

> I had 3,000 to 4,000 baht [about $100 to $130] worth of them; I was selling them and had just run out. My money was in my pocket, and I went to three or four different places that morning after the market, and when I looked in my pocket afterward 1,000 was gone. . . . I wasn't surprised or upset. It was karma. It wasn't a big deal, *mai pen rai* [never mind]. . . . *Tham jai*; I made my heart. I went to go look for more.

A man related a similar kind of feeling when some people swindled him out of his money:

> It happened when I was a youngster—*nuum*—and newly married. "Eighteen Crowns" is the name of the gang who took my money. I sold a lot of

things back then. I had some goods I was going to sell; I had bought them from a business for 3,000 baht and was going to mark them up and sell them. And when I looked at the supply truck that was delivered, that the Eighteen Crowns gang had delivered to me, I opened the boxes and there were just old rags instead of the things I'd ordered. But when I went back to the people who'd sold them they were gone. How do I feel? I'm making my heart.

When I sat down with the head monk in the rural neighborhood of Chang Kao at a little table in his monastery grounds, his hands dirty from the cement wall he was building, I asked him to discuss a time he lost something—what had happened, and how he felt. He said, "Less than a year ago I was on a motorbike and my wallet fell out of my robes. I didn't feel bad, because I let it go [*ploy*]."[2]

A schoolteacher, Somkiet, elaborated on his feelings when he lost money at school:

My working money . . . it was about five or six years ago. Thirty thousand baht! But I told myself, it's something that's happened, it's really happened. This story, this thing, I've let it go, laid it down [*ploy-wang*]. It wasn't my money, it was the money of my office, and I was in charge of looking after it. But I was the one who lost it. So I had to pay it back. I didn't have money, so every month I had to pay a certain amount. It was there, and then "pop!" it wasn't there. *Ploy wang*—I've let it go. I've accepted it, I agreed that it was gone [*yom rap*]. I made my heart.

Aung and I had gone to a wedding in a village near Mae Jaeng one afternoon, and on returning from the festivities Aung looked in her purse and realized that a 1,000-baht note, about 30 U.S. dollars, had apparently fallen out. One thousand baht is not a small amount of money for Aung; each day after slaughtering the pigs she had raised she makes only about

---

2. This monk's story is especially interesting. Usually monks in Thailand neither keep money nor ride motorbikes. If the monk had told me a story about villagers donating money that he then misplaced, or had related another scenario that was more in line with how monks usually are thought to interact officially with money in Thailand, then when he said he let go of the loss I might have thought that he was offering more of a formal presentation of Buddhist philosophy than a personal experience. The fact that he felt comfortable telling me about his motorbike ride and his wallet made me feel that his comment about letting go was less a discursive lesson to me as the visiting American anthropologist, and more an actual affective reaction.

100 baht selling them in the stuffy and smelly room where the meat vendors sell their goods at the market. Her work wasn't easy, and 1,000 baht represented over a week of her earnings. When she realized the loss, I looked at her curiously to see how she felt. She did not look upset, angry, worried, sad, or any of the feelings that I, as her friend, was feeling for her.

"Let's go back and look for it!" I said to her, distressed.

"Never mind," she said, "it's gone. It's OK. I'll find some more money." It was not that she didn't care; she *tham jai*'d. If I didn't know her well, as just a visitor stopping by to interview people, I might not have believed her. But I had known Aung for a while at that point and knew her moods. She wasn't always in a good mood, but this time she was. Later I checked with Sen and Gaew, who had been with us, to see if they read Aung's reaction the same way I had. They concurred that she really was "OK" with the loss. Instead of being angry or sad, when Aung realized she had lost her money, she laughed. It was a kind of laughter I was starting to notice, often accompanying instances that had at first seemed to me to invite a different kind of emotional reaction.

I noticed this emotional orientation in Mae Jaeng often. Once, when the river flooded during the rainy season and homes were ruined, as seemed to happen every year, Sen and I drove to the washed-out bridge. We watched people smiling and talking almost merrily as they pointed out their flooded fields to each other and began repairing the bridge. Aung stopped by, telling us, "Come on, we've got to clean the house or the TV will get ruined!" Sen turned to me and said, "Every year this happens!" The flood would have real, negative implications for the livelihood of people in the area, but the mood felt pleasant. In one perspective, the lighthearted atmosphere seemed to be a way of coping with feelings of loss, but in another it was less a cover for sadness and distress and more a part of letting go and making the heart.

This was the case for personal as well as group problems. When a friend of Gaew's came by the shop house one afternoon to announce that she had just had a miscarriage, she smiled roundly. Even though we knew the pregnancy had meant a lot to her, Gaew smiled too, saying, "It's karma. *Tham jai*. I'm sorry for you." The lightheartedness of the tone was quiet and kind; I was tempted to write in my field notes that night that the smile covered sadness, but that wasn't what was happening. It was not a joking matter to cover up a feeling of sadness, nor even to make light of the situation; and it certainly wasn't that Gaew didn't care. The laughing exchange was a sincere communication of sympathy, a supportive moment to help in letting go of the pregnancy and the dreams of the future that had come with it.

When I became closer with Gaew and Sen, I asked them about their uncle Anurak, who had died in the motorcycle accident that had happened when I first stayed in Mae Jaeng. They told me how they had gotten the news:

"It was the middle of the night when the phone rang," Gaew said. "The head doctor, Moh Bom, was on the other line. I still remember what he first said. He started off with, '*Tham jai dii dii na*' [make your heart well]." She told me that that phrase had started out the experience of learning about her uncle's death and preparing the funeral. Gaew and Sen talked of other things about Uncle Anurak, about how all the karaoke bars in Mae Jaeng were closed down after the accident, and how they still remember trips they had taken with him before the crash. But this idea of *tham jai* seemed to be in the forefront in their minds.

In interviews when I was told about an accident or a death I had heard this idiom of making the heart.

> My parents died about three years ago, from old age. I felt very sad, but I let it go. I accepted it, I *tham jai*'d.

> I had taken care of her, and when she died I was OK.

> My dad died seven years ago. His health was bad, he couldn't breathe. He was seventy-six. The doctor said, "You have to make your heart. Make your heart stable and make merit for your father."

Some people in their interviews even mentioned that Moh Bom had told them this exact piece of advice when he called and prepared them for the news from the hospital. It seemed a little bit like Moh Bom was saying, "I'm about to tell you something difficult." Telling people to "*tham jai*" was seen as a concrete, active practice, and not just an abstracted ideal.

Rituals of Practice: Sand Castles, Floating Boats, Changing Names, and Making Merit

The New Year festival of Songkran is Thailand's most celebrated holiday. It is held during April, the hottest month in an already very warm country. Songkran serves as an exuberant time of renewal, and in Chiang

Mai the revelry is a sight to behold. The streets are packed with thousands and thousands of people throwing, splashing, pouring, and dousing each other with water, often while drunk and usually carrying around giant water guns when they go out, or standing outside of houses with hoses to soak passersby. No one is exempt during Songkran; children douse their elders, people hide in their homes. A newspaper article from Chiang Mai that came out around Songkran said that the city's new Domino's delivery service hit record highs for orders during the week of Songkran, as even going out in public for a few minutes to get food meant getting soaked in seconds.

In Mae Jaeng the celebrations are more subdued, but they are still eventful. Two days before Songkran, Gaew, Goy, and almost everyone else in Mae Jaeng cleaned out their houses and cut their hair. On the first day of Songkran, Gaew and Noi set up a water station outside their shop with buckets and a hose, dousing everyone passing by on foot or motorbike, excepting the really old people, who were *wai*-ed to instead. Sometimes even they weren't immune. Gaew and Noi were soaked from head to foot when I showed up at noon. Their father came out from the shop and joined in the fun for a while, first receiving a proper initial soaking from Noi. Around mid-afternoon, when everyone's hair was shiny and limp from the water, Gaew suddenly announced, "Let's go out around town!" She, Noi, their cousin La, Noi's friend Bom, and I all climbed into the back of the family pickup truck, laughing. Even Sen decided to join, though Gaew looked at him skeptically and a bit surprised when he said he'd be coming with us. By this point Sen rarely left the house, and almost never took part in festivals. She shrugged happily, though, and he got into the driver's seat of the cab, driving around picking up other friends and maneuvering through Mae Jaeng with a big drum full of water in the back of the truck. We threw water from the back of the pickup truck onto people sitting outside their homes, onto each other, onto others passing by in the backs of pickup trucks, while everyone played car stereos at their highest volume. We splashed monks, they splashed us. Only Sen stayed dry behind the wheel, his window closed.

After about an hour or two of driving around the main strips of town we crossed the bridge to the bank of the Mae Jaeng River and, our water tank empty, pulled over to park by dozens of other trucks, where people were getting out to wade in the river. We clambered out of the truck and joined the mass of people moving to the water. Gaew, Aung, and Noi pulled the tank off the truck and waded out to fill it with sand from the river bottom. The drum full again, this time with sand, we got back into the truck and crossed back across the bridge into town, over to the monastery grounds of Wat Kung, our neighborhood monastery, where a *chedi sai*, a sand stupa, was being constructed with the silt from the river. The sand stupa looked like a gigantic sand castle, over fifteen feet tall and ten feet wide, with bright paper banners tucked into all sides. We pulled over and got out, and like the other soaked people around us dumped some sand from the drum onto the enormous castle. A few minutes later we got back in and continued over to Wat Gu, another monastery down the road, and did the same. There the sand castle was even bigger. Just weeks earlier Noi had been living there as a serious, quiet novice monk; now the place seemed discombobulated, with soaking-wet people, both old and young, laughing and celebrating loudly. Two more stops at local monasteries and the sand was all gone, the task done, and we all went home to shower and dry off.

I tried asking Gaew the meaning of the sand castle while we were in the truck driving between the monasteries, but I couldn't get a good answer from her at the time in the chaos; "It's just what we do," she said. "It doesn't have any meaning." When I asked later, though, as we gathered over a meal in the evening, I got a different story: "The sand is the sand from the wat. Every year thousands of people walk into and out of the wat grounds. Their feet carry away the dirt [or sand, as is often found on wat grounds] on the bottoms of their feet. The sand in the castles replenishes it."

Like stories told about desire and attachments in the face of loss, this explanation seemed at first self-contradictory. On one hand it seemed to be an attempt at creating permanence, in terms of putting sand back where it had left, which would reflect the counter-doctrinal opposite of an appreciation for change. But on the other hand it also was a recognition that even in the monastery, impermanence is inevitable. Even the physical structures of the monastery are transitory. I heard other explanations, too, about cosmological orientations in space and footprints in the sand, but the story about the movement of sand from feet to the river and back to the monastery on this day seemed especially poignant. That night, finally showered and dry, I fell asleep thinking about the contradictions of the New Year, as a time for letting go and starting over through an awareness of change.

The "Festival of Lights," called Loy Krathong, is the second-biggest national holiday in Thailand. Loy Krathong is celebrated throughout the country every November and is another striking ritual practice in letting go, even more explicit in this focus than the Thai New Year. It is a time to float away worries. During the three-day festival I went with Gaew and Sen to one of their childhood friend's house up on the nearby mountain. As at virtually all celebrations in Mae Jaeng there was music, whiskey, and plenty of delicious food. Everyone sat outside looking over the valley, listening to music and joking around. As the night wore on, someone brought out large paper lanterns and started assembling them. I had seen these lanterns in the sky by the thousands in Chiang Mai during other trips to Thailand; they had become a kind of cultural tourist symbol of their own. The contraptions are called *loy fai*, floating lanterns, three feet tall with a wick in the center.

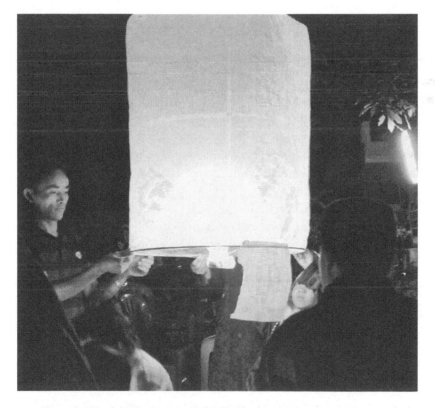

Figure 8. Friends in Mae Jaeng prepare to send burning lanterns into the sky as part of the Loy Krathong festival. Photo by Rosalyn Hansrisuk.

"Hold the lantern up and out in front of you," Gaew instructed, showing me as we gathered around.

"Now light it, and let it go." We let go, and the lantern floated, *loy*, up into the air, a little glowing light disappearing into the night.

"It floats away your thoughts and worries from the year," Gaew explained. We sent a few more out into the sky, watching in silence as the Mae Jaeng valley filled with the lanterns of others doing the same. Late into the night we got back on our motorbikes and into our pickup trucks and drove home. Like so many other occasions in Mae Jaeng, the evening was a mixture of revelry and quietness.

The next morning, Gaew, Aung, and I got ready to go to the town reservoir, a lake near the foothills of Mae Jaeng's surrounding mountains. The reservoir is fed by the mountain above it, providing drinking water to the town. On the south side it continues on as a creek, emptying out into the main Mae Jaeng River. Before leaving, we prepared little *krathong*, or "boats" made of large palm fronds with flowers and a candle inside them.

When we got to the reservoir, we parked and walked over to the water's edge. "You let this go in the river," Aung instructed, as we placed it on the water, "and it floats away your troubles." She used the word *loy* for float, the first word in the name of the holiday. The sentiment of floating away troubles almost repeated word for word what Gaew had told me the night before about the lanterns. In Chiang Mai, the practice is usually done at night, with thousands of small boats crowding the Nam Mae Ping. In Mae Jaeng however, it was a morning activity, and more personal and private. Only a few people were around. "We float the boats together," Aung said, "meaning our lives are moving together."

"I've been feeling too stressed lately," Mae Daeng said when I got home from interviewing one day weeks later and found her sitting on the floor of the living room folding bamboo leaves into the shape of a small boat. She had had a bad cold for a few weeks, and had gone to see Nan Jan, one of Mae Jaeng's two spirit doctors, to see how to get better. She had also gotten some medicine from Ban, who as Mae Jaeng's pharmacist had some biomedical cures to offer; but she still wasn't feeling well.[3] "Nan Jan said to

---

3. "Traditional" herbal or spiritual medicine and "Western" biomedicine are often used concurrently in Mae Jaeng. The main hospital even has an office on its grounds for those seeking massage and other traditional Thai types of cures, and their popularity is growing. For more on

make a *krathong*," she told me, "and float it in the river." Goy and I helped her finish the boat and adorn it with incense and flowers. The three of us walked down to the edge of the river a few blocks from the house, moving aside the brush that had grown up on the shore. Mae Daeng offered a little chant as she placed the boat in the water, and we watched it float away. Both the Songkran Thai New Year and the Loy Krathong festival are large, national events. Much more common are the many smaller, more personal ritual events in people's lives like the one Mae Daeng did on her own. These also, in their own ways and with their own personal meanings, help people practice letting go.

Everyday activities of making merit are especially pronounced; they constitute the core religious activities of the region. People "make merit" when they make offerings in the name of the religion. These offerings most often take the form of money donated to the monastery or gift baskets of toiletries for the monks, but they can take many other forms as well, from ordination to just thinking "good vibes." Virtually everyone in Mae Jaeng makes merit regularly, in some form or another.

Early on in my stay in Mae Jaeng I had learned about merit making from Mae Daeng. The two of us were sitting on the floor of the main monastery building of our neighborhood wat on *wan phra*, the weekly Buddha day where more people go to the wat than usual. Mae Daeng had showed me how to fill a bowl with flowers, incense, candles, and popped rice, all of which she had brought from the house that morning.

"We're making merit," she had said. She modeled for me how to sprinkle the popped rice and wrap the flowers in a bamboo leaf, and line up with the others holding their bowls in front of them as the monks chanted.

"Why are we doing this?" I had asked.

"Because it's good to do. It helps us have good karma in the future. It helps us get the things we want: health for ourselves, our children. . . ."

---

traditional healing and its relationship with biomedicine in Thailand see Puaksom 2007 and Bamber 1998. The Mae Jaeng hospital's local traditional medicine specialist, Padungpon Sukontamontrikul, received his master's degree in traditional medicine at Bangkok's prestigious Mahidol University, rather than following the older, more traditional pattern of learning about local healing from a relative or local healer of an earlier generation. Padungpon's prominence within the hospital, rather than apart from it, points to increasing interconnections among medical practices in the region.

I asked Goy later about making merit as we offered cellophane-wrapped buckets of toothpaste and tissue paper to a monk she had earlier been chatting with casually. "I do it to feel good," she told me. "It helps me feel calm and good, and to practice letting go."

"Making merit doesn't have to mean giving money to the wat," one old man told me. It takes hundreds if not thousands of forms, he said. Offering food to monks counts as making merit, as does offering food and goods, offering one's child to the Sangha, or one's own self in ordination.

"That man makes a lot of merit around here," Sen said in passing as another man left the shop we were sitting in one afternoon. I craned my neck to see the man as he walked away. Sen continued, "He just donated 4,000 baht to the hospital." Donations to the hospital, to the school, to the poor all count as making merit. Ordaining as a monk is especially meritorious. Even ordaining to make merit for one's mother, one of the most commonly cited reasons for ordaining as a novice or a monk in Mae Jaeng, is circumscribed with this idea of giving.

Chai and I were walking down the main road in Mae Jaeng when he stooped to move a little frog that was in the middle of the road. It wasn't stuck there, but it may have been moving too slowly to avoid getting run over by a car. Chai "let it go," moving it over to the side of the road, and laughed, saying, "I've made my merit for the day." He said it half-jokingly, perhaps considering it a silly thing to say, but meaning it. His behavior and his stated reason were similar to a practice common to the heavily visited wats in Chiang Mai, where, for a small fee, vendors will make money by helping people make merit: the visitors pay to free small birds from cages, letting the birds go and making merit for themselves in the process. The birds have been trained to come right back to the cage, and this is no secret for the customer, but that's hardly important; it is the symbolic act of letting something go that creates the merit. It is both the symbolism of the action and the action itself that make the merit; it is the intentional feeling that does the work.

"Let's say you donate something to the wat," Gaew said when I asked her to explain more about merit, "but you're in a bad mood when you do it, and you don't want to do it—you just throw it in the donation bowl in a huff; in that case you didn't actually make any merit at all. It's not the things that matters, it's the feeling. You have to feel calm, and good, and want to give." It's not the action per se that counts, but the feeling of giving that is felt while engaging in the practice.

This emphasis on the affective aspect of merit is central to the act: "If you go up to a monk and give him something but you don't really want to do it," I was told by an old man in an interview, "if you don't feel like making an offering, like you're in a bad mood ..." The man paused to illustrate, mimicking pushing something toward someone gruffly, with eyes averted. "What do you think, is that making merit? No! You don't get merit from that." Others who were crowded around him to listen to the interview nodded in agreement.

Generally speaking, the sentiment in Mae Jaeng surrounding merit is about feeling and intention. A woman I spoke with summed this up nicely when she said, "Making merit is about doing anything good that's done with a giving intention." This seems like merit making could refer to virtually anything, and indeed this is how it is taken. In Mae Jaeng, religious practices as a whole incorporate nonattached, positive intentions of giving, and letting go.[4]

Gender and Power: Is Letting Go a Gendered and Hierarchical Ideal?

Training of nonattachment through letting go is a shared ideal in Mae Jaeng, but it isn't something that everyone does equally, or equally well. One evening during a town festival I came by Gaew's shop to find her

---

4. There are many activities happening around Mae Jaeng that have religious connotations, with the many influences that could each be labeled more or less "Buddhist"; yet people rarely label things as more or less "Buddhist." Even the spirit doctors with their astrological charts and esoteric chants are referred to with the prefix "Nan," an honorific term meaning that one used to be a Buddhist monk. Ritual activities almost always have multiple meanings. In highlighting the attention they draw to impermanence I do not mean to suggest that other meanings are not also at play. Among many other purposes, for example, the Northern Thai practice of tying the white strings of *sai sin* around one's wrists (and wats and new vehicles) is understood to ward off ghosts and gather together one's soul or wits (*khwan*), as well as to help not feeling too stressed (Eberhardt 2006). Banners flown at funerals are understood to help the deceased rise to the heavens, as well as serve as reminders of impermanence and the inevitability of death (Hall 2008). The *chedi sai* at the New Year (and a similar but smaller Northern Thai ritual Sang Wihan Chamlong) has been explained as a way to replenish the grains of sand that people took away but weren't theirs to take (Rajadhon 1986, 182) and as a way that "people who can't afford to build a monastery building gain merit by building this [free] one," as Sen told me, as well as being a reminder of change. And the boats floated at the Loy Krathong festival have also been used for offerings to departed ancestors, and to appease the spirit of an ancient monk named Upagupta, in addition to floating away worries (Swearer 2010).

managing the desk while the rest of her family were out enjoying themselves at the celebration. Mae Jaeng has only a few nighttime events; usually by 8 or 9 p.m. the town is almost completely silent. On this night, though, a rare nighttime festival was taking place. It was the annual *tin jok* cloth festival, the festival for which Goy had joined the planning committee and then left. People had come to celebrate from all over Northern Thailand, and some even from as far away as Bangkok. At 10 p.m. the main road was still crowded with festivalgoers. Mae San and Paw Nui were running a ring-toss booth that was raising money for the Red Cross; Noi was running around with his schoolmates; Sen was nowhere to be seen, probably at Chai's house. Gaew's shop was only five hundred meters from the main intersection where the festival was being held, and when I went in to say hello I found her there alone. People were wandering in with friends, buying beer and chatting as they headed out again.

I sat down with Gaew to talk; she was smiling and laughing too, but I could tell she was out of sorts. She didn't say anything much about it, and when I asked how she was doing she said she was good. After a while she said casually, "Everyone else is out there having fun . . . but I have to mind the store." I could see she wanted to go and was struggling a bit with not desiring to. She didn't seem angry, or frustrated, or even upset as such; all these represent emotions that were too agitated or articulated (even unconsciously) to correctly describe her state of mind. But there was something I felt I recognized as the beginning of a feeling of frustration. It was one that Gaew worked on at that point, to turning an itchy feeling of restlessness into an emotion of comfort and acceptance. She even laughed when she told me about the others out having fun. It was a laugh I got used to over time, the same kind of laugh people had when looking at their flooded fields, a laugh that had first felt unnerving, even false, when emotions didn't seem to match what I was used to from people I knew back home in similar circumstances. It may be this unnerving feeling that makes anthropologists start to question assumptions about psychological universalism and diversity, when people they study seem to feel in ways that don't at first make sense; when they dance instead of cry at funerals, when "sadness" is presumed to be experienced the same everywhere, and the anthropologist (for example, Rosaldo 1984, Shweder et al. 2008, Geertz 1960) realizes that it really is not.

I sat with Gaew for a while, and eventually other friends joined us, turning the shop itself into an extension of the street festival. I thought about how I had rarely seen Gaew seem sad or sullen. I realized that most of the time she was really good at letting go of things; she accepted things the way they were, if not immediately then over time. I recalled the time I had come by her shop and vented about having to leave Mae Daeng's house, or the time I had gotten upset when Ari kept showing up late, and I had complained to her. She had listened and empathized but mostly thought my behavior odd, even "foreign." No wonder my emotions had seemed so childish and incompetent to her; I was attached to things not the way they were, but the way I wanted them to be. Gaew clearly had a desire to take part in the festival that night, but she didn't seem especially upset about it, or at least not as upset as I would imagine she would be. She wasn't just putting on a front of not being sad, either. She told me she was OK with the situation, and I could only conclude that she really did feel that way.

I thought of Gaew's feelings as I walked home down the main drag of town that night, surrounded by people celebrating. I also wondered why she had to stay alone minding the shop while her brother was out with his friends, her husband was out with his friends, and even her parents and her little brother were enjoying themselves. I realized that Gaew seemed to do more than the others in the household: not only did she manage the store more than the rest of the family; she also had a side business selling car insurance, and she did almost all the cleaning and washing for the household.

Many feminist anthropologists I admire point out the ways that power and privilege make their way into the social expectations that people have of each other (Butler 1999; Lutz and Abu-Lughod 1990; Ortner 1997). Since these scholars have shown that women are so often the losers in conservative cultural practices, I wondered if my growing awareness of acceptance and nonattachment was just highlighting norms that served to perpetuate a gendered social order that disenfranchised half the population.

When Mae Daeng had gone to her yearly weeklong meditation retreat a few weeks earlier at a cave monastery in the mountains near Mae Jaeng, and I went with her, I had seethed every day at mealtime as I and the other women there made the midday meal for the male meditators, who for their part sat comfortably eating the fruit of the women's labor. Mae Daeng hadn't complained, and when I asked her about it after, she dismissed my contention as unimportant; but seeing Gaew mind the shop and watching her come to terms with what appeared to be gendered labor inequalities, I started to wonder more about gender and other social hierarchies in emotional practices related to the conceptions of calmness, making the heart, and letting go.

Two hypotheses seemed plausible to explain what hierarchical social differences look like in Buddhist emotional practices. One suggests social superiors will be more emotional than juniors, and the other suggests they will be less so. On the one hand it might be suspected that those in more powerful positions would have more leeway to experience and express whatever emotions they felt like, with those in more junior, inferior positions on the social ladder required to be more submissive and quiet, with the expectation that they rein in their emotions.[5] On the other hand, those in more powerful positions might be seen as more responsible and able to control their emotions, with those lower on the social ladder less stoic and more likely to feel and express emotions, and be more "emotional." These may be two prominent though opposite stereotypes at play in the U.S. context of emotion and social hierarchy, but neither seemed clearly the case in Mae Jaeng.

Gaew laughed off my question when I asked her the day after the festival about gendered emotion and the expected moral behaviors of different people. School had just let out in town, and she, Sen, and I were sitting together in the shop selling gum and candy to little kids in their school uniforms coming through with their parents on their way home. We talked about what kinds of behaviors were seen as the mark of a "good" person in Mae Jaeng, and what kinds of behaviors were seen as "bad."

"Like, if someone stays up late at night, that's bad, right?" I asked.

"Yeah."

"What about if they sleep in?" I was thinking of Mae Daeng getting up at the crack of dawn, or before, to go to the market to start selling goods, and how sometimes, rising as I usually did at the apparently late hour of 7 a.m., I would be deemed a bit of a slacker.

"No, sleeping in is OK," Gaew said.

---

5. This is the position advocated, for example, in Unni Wikan's *Managing Turbulent Hearts*, in regard to emotion and social hierarchy on the nearby Southeast Asian island of Bali (1990).

Sen at first nodded but then paused and disagreed: "Well, if you're male it's OK to sleep in. But if you're female that's bad."

"What! Why?"

"Well, women have to do a lot—they have to cook and work and do everything. So it's bad if they don't get up early."

Sen seemed to be re-creating exactly the kind of gender inequality I feared. But as he continued, his reason seemed to turn things around: "It's because the women are in charge here. The men, well, look around you, they don't do anything. This is a town of women, for women. Look at all the things that have the word "mother" in them: *Mae* [mother] is in everything—the name of the town Mae Jaeng, the river Mae Nam Mae Jaeng, Mae . . . everything! In central Thailand it's different . . . like with the king—when he dies pretty much everyone wants the princess to be the new ruler, but it won't happen, because down there women can't be rulers of the kingdom. But up here we've had women rulers, in Haripunjai there was the queen. . . . The only reason women aren't allowed to be monks," he continued, "is that the men around here want something for themselves. Because otherwise the women would overrun this town."

Sen and I turned to Gaew: did she agree that women were the leaders in Mae Jaeng? She nodded in the affirmative, smiling: "Uh-huh."

I told Mae Daeng about Sen's comments later and asked if she agreed with him. She laughed and nodded affirmatively, too: "Yes, women are in charge here."

Goy was usually in charge of things, even in relation to higher-status men she interacted with; I recalled her walking around with her microphone during community events, practically ordering a senior monk once on what to do during a temple festival. It was clearly the case that Goy was more powerful in relation to her brother Ta, though Ta was a bit "off" and so not very representative of others. But Goy was not just in charge of her house; she was often in charge in situations involving men of higher status. People talked about the house I lived in as Mae Daeng's house, or as Goy's house; they never referred to it as Ta's. The house and shop that Sen and Gaew lived in followed a similar, female-gendered line; it was called their mother Mae San's place, not their father's. Before that it was known as their grandmother Mon's. Some people were starting to refer to it now as Gaew's, never as Sen's, or Noi's, or Gaew's husband Pan's. Their father Paw Nui didn't seem as central to the activities of the family, and neither did Pan, Sen, or Noi. Sen even told me that sometimes he drank alcohol because he didn't have anything else to do. He and Noi and Paw Nui helped out at the shop sometimes, but they were not central to it. Gaew or her mom made all the financial decisions, and almost all other decisions, too. It wasn't just the household that women seemed to be in charge of either, as if powerful only in the inner sanctum, as has been described for women's domains in other cultures like India or Indonesia, with men ruling the social world outside. Women in Mae Jaeng are very much a part of the social public, walking, driving, and doing errands around town, selling and buying goods at the market, taking part in government activities, trading activities, religious activities, and sporting events, and even drinking and "hanging out" in mixed gender groups in the evenings. Women hold positions of power at the wat, organizing events and festivals and spoken to deferentially even by head monks. Men are often blamed for failings at home and business, and they often blame themselves, but I had heard neither a man blame a woman for their problems nor my woman friends complain that men had done so.

The traditional matrilineal thread of movement between households in Northern Thailand may have something to do with this relative power of women in the area. When I first arrived at Mae Daeng's house she had introduced her family and told me that her nine brothers and sisters all lived within a few blocks.

"And what about your husband's family?" I had asked her.

"Oh, he comes from Chiang Dao. He doesn't have any family here."

I didn't think much of this until I heard that Pan, Gaew's husband, was also from another town, Chom Thong, and was living in her family's house. I started asking around, and it turned out that for almost all couples I knew, the husband and wife lived close to the wife's family, or the husband took up residence in the family household itself. I recalled reading in an ethnography that it was traditional for men in Northern Thailand to move into the wife's home, but until I saw it happening for people I knew, I had missed the implications of the practice. In India most young brides take up residence in their husband's home and re-create themselves according to those rules (Jessor, Colby, and Shweder 1996; Menon and Shweder 1998), and in a similar but oppositely gendered way, men in Mae Jaeng find themselves in an unsettling foreign environment when they move as new grooms into their wife's home.

"Yeah, I miss my parents," Pan told me one day; "they're in Chom Thong. I'd like to build them a new house there one day. I visit as much as I can, but I'm so busy...." Pan had married Gaew only a few years earlier, and I could see that his attachments to his old life were still strong, but he was reconstituting himself in his new home. Pan worked at the public health center in town, coming home only for lunch and later in the evenings. In Gaew's house he was still an outsider; his place in the household was a far second to that of his wife.

Rather than feelings, it was more often behaviors that were labeled as especially "male" or "female." One night, Mae Daeng was wheeling into the bathroom a heavy gas canister that would give us hot water for showers. As I came over to help, she looked up at me with sweat on her face and said, laughing and nodding to the container, "With my husband gone I have to be the woman *and* the man in this house!"

While talking with her another night about how I found Sen's cooking to be second only to Mae Daeng's herself, she unexpectedly told me, "Yeah, well, when he was a teenager Sen was a *kathoey*," referring to a third gender category used in Thai for effeminate males.[6] "He used to wear earrings and everything," she went on, "but now he's more of a man." She was suggesting that it is a man's job to lift heavy things, and that cooking or wearing earrings are things women do. But comments like hers seemed to suggest that while behaviors may be gendered, feelings, and even bodies, are less so.[7] It was through his actions rather than his feelings that Sen became more male.

Maybe gender was not a prominent factor in the expectations and experiences of letting go and related emotional practices for people I knew;

---

6. The popularity of a *kathoey* identity (a third-gender category considered by people I knew in Thailand to have come from India) is transitioning in contemporary Thailand to the idea of the gay male identity (as fully male but attracted to men, considered to come from the United States). For more on changing issues of sexuality in Thailand see Kāng 2012; Boonmongkon and Jackson 2012; Wilson 2004; Jackson 1989; Sinnott 2004; Dicks 2006; Fuhrmann 2009.

7. To find out more about attitudes toward gender and bodies, I asked people in Mae Jaeng whether they thought it was strange if someone changed his or her gender. I was surprised when over half the respondents indicated that this was not a strange thing at all. They often linked their explanations to nature; as one man told me, "It's natural for people to change their gender, because our gender reflects the hormones inside of us. It's our hearts, it's nature. It's the nature of the heart. It's the body that doesn't correlate, it's the body, say, of a man, but the heart is of a woman, it's their nature. So the outside is just changing with the natural inside."

but it occurred to me that I had perhaps inadvertently fallen in with a particularly "feminist" group of people in Mae Jaeng. Maybe their attitudes did not reflect those of the community more broadly, which might have different expectations of gender stereotypes and emotion. I looked systematically through my interviews to see if there were differences in emotional responses between genders. But although I noted descriptions of things that men did and things that women did, I found little in the way of affective differences; the interviews reinforced rather than contradicted the conclusions about emotionality that I was coming to from more casual observation.

In talking about women's responsibilities, in one sense Sen was re-creating the problematic popular Thai discourse of the powerful woman as the "hind legs" of the "elephant," the driving force behind her man. Culturally constructed gender roles between males and females in Mae Jaeng put women at a disadvantage in several senses: the fact that women cannot ordain into the powerful and respected community of monks is the most prominent of them.[8] There was only one *mae chee* (a Buddhist nun) in Mae Jaeng; even in the broader national Thai context where *mae chee* are relatively rare, the fact of there being only one *mae chee* is especially unusual for an area overflowing with male monks and novices.

When I asked one of Mae Daeng's nieces where her husband was, whom I had heard about but never met, she replied vaguely that he was away. Later it was mentioned to me in gossip that maybe her husband had another wife, and I was reminded that a Thai concept called *mia noi* (mistress, or literally, "little wife") is a felt part of life for some in Mae Jaeng.

"Women uphold morality," I was told more than once, and the other side of women upholding morality suggested that men in comparison do not. Women as the upholders of morality suggests that men were freer to break with moral virtues, and Sen's statement seemed to reiterate it. Feminist scholars have argued that Thai Buddhist ideals of desire are gendered in practice: women and especially representations of women and desire in different cultural contexts are seen as especially tumultuous, and hence dangerous (Bowie 2011, 2008; Fuhrmann 2009). Marjorie Muecke

---

8. Female monkhood is not recognized by the official Thai Sangha (based on an edict from 1928), but attitudes toward female ordination are slowly changing, and a few women, led by the venerable Bhikkhuni Dhammananda, have decided to ordain regardless of official recognition.

describes one of the repercussions of this inequality in the case of a form of distress in Thailand called "wind illness," a culturally localized Thai mental health disorder: "Ethnographic evidence suggests that 'wind illness' may be a somatization of stress," Muecke says, "again particularly among the poor, but also among women. In general in Thai society men are permitted more ways to relieve tension and escape social responsibilities than women. Men may enter the monkhood, gaining social status as well as sanction for leaving their normal responsibilities aside. . . . Society in general puts more domestic responsibility on women and provides them with fewer escapes than it does men" (1979, 291).

Some of the issues that Muecke describes are present in Mae Jaeng, among them the domestic responsibility of women and the exclusivity of monkhood for men. But the gendered emotional landscape in Mae Jaeng looks quite different from the one Muecke describes, or that a diachronic gender analysis might suggest. Although in one sense Sen was re-creating an excuse of power that masked actual inequality in women's roles when he told me that women had to wake up early and work harder because they are in charge, he was also making a different point, one that did put women at a higher status. By referencing Queen Camadevi, the seventh-century female ruler of an area that is now in Northern Thailand (Indrawooth 1999), and circumscribing the monkhood as the singular attempt at power from the otherwise powerless male population, Sen was suggesting that women were expected to work harder not because they are the inferiors but because they are the leaders. It put women at the forefront, the "front legs of the elephant" even, rather than at the back of social life in Mae Jaeng.

In Mae Jaeng women control the money and work alongside men in the fields planting and harvesting;[9] they govern the transaction of goods and take part in government, and even (very arguably), they also perpetuate the Sangha, the Buddhist community: while only men can ordain, and the wat and its powerful members may seem dominated by men, the women in Mae Jaeng often ran the show even there, too, organizing events, visiting their young ordained sons, and making decisions about the monks'

---

9. As paid labor is becoming more common in Northern Thailand, rather than the system of shared work cycling through the valley's fields in neighborhood harvesting parties, this equality of women is being threatened: according to the standard rate in Mae Jaeng, female laborers earn two-thirds as much as their male counterparts.

activities. The domain of the Sangha as a powerful mark of inequality is not a small issue, and social movements to promote female monastic ordinations are growing; but women in many ways really are the most powerful gender in Mae Jaeng. Contrary to my expectations, I found no marked gender difference in the kinds of emotions that people reported having or being expected to have. When people did have emotional problems, their gender sometimes was referenced; but from what I could tell, there was not a fixed and gendered double standard of emotionality. Such a finding, or lack of one, challenges a long history of scholarship that suggests that Thai women are disadvantaged in their expected emotions compared with men.

Gender may be relatively insignificant for socially expected differences in affective comportment, but interpersonal hierarchy is very important in Thai life, and gender is inscribed within this. The social world in Mae Jaeng, as in all of Thailand, is hyper-stratified and hierarchical. Friends preface each other's name with *P'* or *Ai'* (elder) and *nong* (younger) according to their relative ages; I would refer to Goy as P'Goy, and Goy in turn would refer to me as Nong Julia; Gaew and I similarly called Sen "P'Sen" and referred to other close, older friends the same way. Unequal hierarchies of respect are implied in these titles, and they can be felt in even the smallest differences in status. Mae Daeng was born five minutes before her twin Mae U, and even for these two relatively most equal of people, Mae Daeng was seen as the older sibling and therefore was marked as deserving more respect. It was a source of eternal mirth for Sen (and no doubt of some consternation, too) that people would sometimes stop by his house and ask him where his sister "P'Gaew" was, using the term to suggest that she was older than he and not realizing that he in fact was the elder. Such blending and blurring of honorifics show that the social status of interpersonal hierarchy is not fixed, but nevertheless it was almost always commented on when broken.

Social hierarchies are felt within the interpersonal space in which emotion is constructed; being aware of others means not just attending to their expectations but also being considerate of the other person's feelings, and the effects of one's feelings in the co-construction of another's. The interpersonal quality of emotion that is not just based off others' feelings but also their expectations within the social, hierarchical world is part of the making of the heart and letting go, as well as the coolness of a *jai yen*.

The Thai phrase *kreng jai* captures this interpersonal hierarchical affective situation well: *kreng jai* is usually translated directly into English as feeling "scared" or "awestruck," but the language of awe or deference misses the interpersonal quality of respect. One feels deferential out of respect to others when one feels *kreng jai*. Anything other than letting go and feeling a *jai yen* is, in a way, considered a selfish act, because, I was told, it pulls others' feelings out of focus, and draws others' emotions into disruption. *Kreng jai* is often thought by scholars to reflect hierarchical social inequalities in which the subordinate is expected to "rein in" his or her (but usually her) emotions, while the senior interlocutor can do whatever he or she (but usually he) feels, and to some extent this hierarchical reading of *kreng jai* rings true in Mae Jaeng. There is a touch of distance in the feeling of *kreng jai*: one would not feel *kreng jai* in the presence of, say, one's younger brother, but one would with an in-law. Even one's parents, because of their higher status, evoke this kind of deferential feeling. Months after the *tin jok* festival, I was talking with Sen about his increasing problems, and he told me that he sometimes wanted to discuss things with his mother but was hesitant to do so because he didn't want to burden her: "I feel *kreng jai*," he said.

This deferential feeling is part of almost all hierarchical interpersonal exchanges in Thailand; and almost all interpersonal exchanges are hierarchical. The most common place that the idea of *kreng jai* comes out is where one is a guest in another's home. When entering an acquaintance's home, one is inevitably told by the congenial host, "Please don't feel *kreng jai*."[10] It is a sentiment similar to saying "make yourself at home," and by being so directed the utterance itself draws attention in a sense to the fact that indeed one *should* feel *kreng jai* in the situation. The usual consequence is to feel *kreng jai* even more strongly. Even after an invitation to not feel *kreng jai* is voiced by my hosts I observed the same kinds of formalities I would have otherwise. When I asked Gaew if she felt this was the case, that one still felt *kreng jai* even when directly told not to, she laughed and said, "Yeah, definitely!" When people are closer with each other than mere acquaintances, however, feelings of *kreng jai* subside. After insisting for months on teaching Gaew English in exchange for the Thai she was helping me with, Gaew

---

10. For more on *kreng jai* see Burnard and Naiyapatana 2004 and Knutson et al. 2003.

finally told me, "Actually, I'm so busy, I don't really want to learn English so much. I was learning because I felt *kreng jai* to you." I was surprised; in this case her statement was a mark that we were now closer friends, but it caused me to become more sensitive to this affective practice in her and others. It is here that the "letting go" of Gaew's earlier wish, perhaps to spend her time in ways other than learning English, reflects a hierarchy that she (at least at first) felt to me as the slightly older and foreign visitor.

It may be the case that Gaew was relegated to managing the shop the night of the festival while others were out because of the double-edged, gendered expectation of being in charge of things and therefore more responsible; but it may also be because of lower status in the social hierarchy of the household in general. In Mae Jaeng parents, elders, and others at a higher social position appear neither more nor less emotional in interactions with their social inferiors. It is possible that, as with gender, those who are more powerful are given more leeway to feel and talk about emotions; but they may also be expected more than others to be able to practice the emotions of letting go and "making the heart."[11] Mae Daeng, Mae San, and Paw Nui did seem more at ease to stretch out and relax at their house than did their children, and in Goy's house Mae Daeng was more likely to tell Ta or me to be quiet than we were to tell each other, or her; but these differences in social hierarchy were small, and especially when my immediate newness had faded and I became more a part of the household, there seemed to be less rather than more structural and gendered differences in emotion.

Emotional expectations to "let go" are inscribed within these sometimes gendered and always hierarchical arenas of social life. In her book *Meditation in Modern Buddhism* (2010), the anthropologist Joanna Cook writes about a year she lived as an ordained nun at a monastery in Chiang Mai: at one point Cook's mother came to visit, and when her mother left, Cook felt "close to tears" (127) while saying goodbye at the airport, already missing her. Afterward, Cook was (kindly) chastised by the other ordained monks and nuns she lived with, who reminded her that Buddhist teachings emphasize the importance of detachment and letting go. At the end of her time in the monastery, however, as she herself was departing at the Chiang Mai airport, Cook tells us that the head monk of the monastery shed a tear when he saw

---

11. Scholars of Thai social dynamics have pointed out that bosses and teachers often think of themselves as moral/spiritual examples for their employees or students (e.g., Wilson 2004).

her off; unlike hers, his emotional act went without comment. "His monastic role was much more," she relates, "than one impermanent emotional expression." When I read her book I took the passage to suggest that the head monk was socially permitted to feel attached to Cook even as Cook wasn't allowed to feel attached to her mother; it seemed that a significant reason for the difference was their differences in power and gender. It seemed to fall to some people more than others to do more of the work of letting go. Yet when I talked with Cook at a conference on Thai studies during a trip to Bangkok and asked her about what I had first read to be centrally an issue of gender and status in her description, of the unequal responses to her own and her head monk's tears, she told me that I was incorrect. It wasn't that the monk was somehow permitted to be attached emotionally while she wasn't. Instead, it was understood that the head monk at her monastery was much more spiritually advanced, and as such his emotional expression was not seen to be as connected to demeritorious attachment. While gender and hierarchy may always be inscribed within religious practices, Cook's explanation reiterates that they are part of larger socially shared Buddhist ideas about practicing letting go and their consequences for interpersonal emotional behavior. The answer to gendered and other power differences may not be an either-or one: men may be symbolically superior in theory, while in social life women call the shots; or the breakdown of power in the gender order may be even more subtle, landing on neither side of the debate, breaking down instead in different ways and in more diverse contexts than a universalizing view of power dynamics might suggest. As a graduate of a women's college and a self-proclaimed feminist, I wanted to see the inequalities that I was taught to attend to; but while inequalities having to do with gender are clearly evident in practice, I did not see them in ways that clearly patterned what I might have expected, especially in the realm of an emotional ideal of detachment. The shared goals and practices of letting go are evident for everyone, as part of larger social dynamics at play.

Letting Go in a World of Change

Attending to letting go (as focused on nonattachment) helps to make sense of otherwise difficult-to-understand behaviors and experiences in the course of everyday life in Buddhist Thailand, not just in Mae Jaeng.

Charles Keyes (1985) offers one such example when he describes a woman called Mrs. K in Northeastern Thailand who was grief-stricken by the death of her mother. After the villagers construct a large bell tower in the center of the village and perform a rite that, we are told, helps the souls of the deceased progress to a new incarnation, she feels better. Keyes explains that it is the ritual action *qua* ritual action that helps. He suggests that rituals and rites everywhere help people to deal with grief at loss. A year after the rite, Keyes tells us, Mrs. K is flourishing. But why a rite to send the soul of Mrs. K's mother on, and not another rite? Maybe any rite would have worked, but people chose this one. Keyes tells us that as the souls of the deceased were able to progress to a new incarnation, they would be "troubled no longer." Paying attention to the role of attachment in ideas about well-being helps to make sense of why. As for most untimely deaths in Thailand, the souls of the deceased are "not yet ready for rebirth"; they continue to have attachments to the living, and the living to them. The souls of the deceased and the mind of Mrs. K were tied up together. In the interpersonal construction of affect (interpersonal even after death), Mrs. K was creating emotions that were attached to her mother. The rite worked because in effect it released Mrs. K's mental bond and "allowed" her mother to continue on; it also "allowed" Mrs. K herself to let go of her attachment.

Nancy Eberhardt (2006) relates a similar incident of loss in a Shan village in Northern Thailand in which a young woman named Nang and her daughter Ying were killed in a lightning storm. Nang's family and friends were fearful of feelings of attachment to the deceased, and it played out in their emotions. Eberhardt tells us that Nang's niece would not say "I am sad" at the passing, but "I feel pity for them," a sentiment that indicates less emotional attachment on behalf of the speaker to the deceased. People told me about attachments to the dead often in interviews. They usually explained the danger as the dead's attachment to the living. But the danger is twofold: it is also the fear of attachments of the living to the dead. Mourning rituals in Thailand work to help detach emotional feelings, thereby "letting" the attachment one has to a loved one "go."

This letting go can be found even in activities that seem on the surface not related at all. One afternoon well into my time in Mae Jaeng I showed up at Gaew and Sen's shop, and neither of them was around. "Where are Gaew and Sen?" I asked their mom after greeting her with palms together in front of me in a Thai *wai*. It was unusual to find both Gaew and Sen away from the shop at the same time in the middle of the day, as usually one of them was on hand to help manage the store. "They're at the head district office," she told me, pointing to the administrative center of town a few hundred meters in front of us. I found the siblings there sitting in chairs waiting to be called up to the front desk.

"Mom told us to change our names," Gaew said, laughing when I asked what was going on. "Mom's already changed hers, and Noi went with her this morning. We're here to change ours, too."

"Why?" I asked. I felt silly asking, aware that I still knew so little about things people around me took for granted, like a child just learning about the world.

Sen looked at me sheepishly and shrugged, bemused. Gaew said, "Well . . . we've been having bad luck lately in our family. The shop isn't doing so well, we're all getting sick. We're doing this to change our fortune."

Gaew showed me the new name she had chosen for herself: Wattana, meaning "prosperity." She went up to the desk when her name was called and came back with a new legal ID card bearing her new name.

Sen followed suit, coming back with Monkut, "crown." "But only," he told me by way of explanation, "because my mom said to, and not for any other reason." I was starting to notice little strange things that Sen did differently from others, either disagreeing with or, more often, not really internalizing practices around him, though his drinking wasn't yet becoming a major problem.

Changing names brings good luck for many reasons, and one of them is the act of nonattachment and letting go of one's identifying label. "Oh, yeah—Goy's name was changed three times," Mae Daeng told me when I asked. "She was sick as a baby, so her uncle suggested it." When I looked into it I found that others changed their names, too. Like so many other everyday rituals in Mae Jaeng, the practice of name changing is not explicitly religious, nor labeled so as particularly Buddhist, but monks are almost always involved in the process. Gaew had shown me a piece of paper at the district office when she changed her name, containing about a dozen names on it: "I chose Wattana from this list the monk at the wat gave me," she said. "The list has all the possible names that start with the right letter that the monk says corresponds with my birth day." Formal names are understood to have cosmological significance in Northern Thailand;

monks are usually consulted, as they were by Gaew and Sen, to suggest auspicious possibilities. Like so many other activities in Mae Jaeng, changing one's name has layered and complex meanings. It was connected to ideas about place, past, and future, and about nonattachment.[12]

Part of practicing nonattachment is about a particular way of thinking about emotion. A schoolteacher I spoke with told me about how he felt when he heard his mother had passed away:

> I was talking with a friend at the school here, about death and about that kind of thing, and while we were talking my sister called to tell me that our mother had died. We were talking about death, and the idea of death, and I was so surprised I couldn't do anything, I didn't have any strength, my knees gave out and I had to sit down quickly. I was close to shock for about a minute, and I sat for a minute of concentration meditation, concentrating on breathing. I was in a condition outside of time. I thought of how impermanence is in our lives for every person, and every person will have experience with it. It's not about religion or country. It's in every step, for everyone. We have to *ploy*, we have to *wang*—to let go of things.

Here letting go and its opposite, attachment, help to make sense of emotional life through an attention to change. The teacher thought of impermanence, and let go of his affective attachment. One of Goy's favorite Buddhist scholars, the famous Thai monk Buddhadasa Bhikkhu, liked to talk about a relationship between sensations and the desires that can become attached to them. On Goy's suggestion I visited Buddhadasa's monastery in Southern Thailand for a meditation retreat, and during a dhamma talk there a monk used the metaphor of a bee sting to illustrate

---

12. The name changing discussed here refers to formal names. Informal names are even less stable and more susceptible to change. Play names (in Thai *chuu len*), as opposed to formal names, are the everyday ones used with friends, such as "Goy" or "Gaew." Friends or family give each other their play names to represent childhood characteristics or sounds the person made as a baby, or cute animals or English words, or personality or circumstantial qualities. The play name of Gaew's friend Ban, for example, literally means "wide," to refer to his wide girth; "Gaew" comes from the Thai for "glass." Gaew's friend was named Rot (car) because she was born in the car on the way to the hospital in Chiang Mai. Sen was named after the infant formula brand "Sen" that he drank as an infant at his grandmother's house instead of breast feeding from his mom. Play names are informal, multiple, and often change, too, over time. They, along with the many indirect words for "I" in the Thai language, also reflect attention to nonattachment to self. But formal name changes take on a deeper cosmological, even religious meaning.

this connection. "Let's say a bee stings you," he said, "and the bee sting feels unpleasant. It is not expected that, even if you were enlightened, you would not experience a feeling of pain. But beyond that feeling you also wish for the feeling to go away; you become attached to that wish, and that brings suffering." Pain (as well as all kinds of unpleasant discomforts, and even pleasant comforts too) is felt and experienced; it is the attachment to these sensations that is harmful.[13] And the reverse, letting go of attachments, promotes well-being.[14] Implicitly and explicitly, successfully and unsuccessfully, the process of crafting calmness through the letting go of attachments is a way that people in Mae Jaeng practice training the mind.

The reason that attachment brings suffering is tied to *anicca*, the idea that everything will change. Nonattachment in this sense is understood to be less an always-imperfect ideal and more a practical orientation that reflects, and cultivates, an ability to attend to, and be aware of, change.[15] When I asked at the end of each interview for reflections on *anicca*, people talked about letting go as part of becoming aware of change:

> [*Anicca*] teaches that we shouldn't grasp things, that we shouldn't hold on to or attach to things. *Ploy*, I let go. . . .

---

13. This attachment may be what in English is thought of as emotion. The Sri Lankan Theravada studies scholar Padmasiri De Silva in his *Introduction to Buddhist Psychology* offers a similar analysis: "With the emergence of craving and grasping, we discern the transition from the state of a feeling into the experience of an emotion" ([1979] 2000, 40). De Silva marks this theory of affect as particular to Buddhism: "[The] ethical and spiritual dimension that cuts across the analysis of feeling, making subtle distinctions between different qualitative levels of pleasure, is of course something alien to modern western psychology" (41).

14. The importance of nonattachment is one of the most prominent topics of Buddhist texts. Like Western psychological views on attachment it often focuses on interpersonal relations. Both the Western psychological perspectives of attachment and Buddhist perspectives focus on intersubjective relations, but while the popular Western psychological model is a developmental model based on the idea of positive "healthy" and negative "unhealthy" attachments that people have to others (Bowlby 1973, 1980, [1969] 1983), in Buddhist accounts attachment is seen as overwhelmingly unhealthy and refers more experientially to desire (for an object, a person, thing, or idea) and the emotions resulting from attaching one's feelings to an object. For more on cross-cultural research on attachment behaviors see Quinn and Mageo 2013 and Sahdra, Shaver, Brown 2010.

15. "Attending to" impermanence in the sense of being aware or mindful of it is seen as good, but I was told by informants that, almost paradoxically, paying too much attention to impermanence in the sense of fixating on it is bad and represents clinging, hence suffering: "If you think about *anicca* all the time," I was told by one, "you're grasping at it, like a taut string, and you don't really understand it."

Life is uncertain. It's *anicca*. Things come and go. If you attach to something, you suffer. I think of it all the time. *Plong*, I lay it down, all the time, because things are not certain.[16]

Anicca is in the lives of every person, and every person will have experience with it. . . . It's in every step, for everyone. We have to *ploy*, we have to *wang*. Let go of things.

A friend in Mae Jaeng related the affective practice of letting go to an awareness of change the following way: A relationship he had been in had just ended; his ex had started seeing someone new, and he said, "I saw the new couple walking by together, and I could see the anger coming toward me, but I thought, "People come and go. Everything changes, so why let it bother me? And I let it go." He was pointing to change as a reason for letting go, and awareness of change as informing his ability to do so. The process can be instantaneous or drawn out, but an awareness of impermanence helps one to make the heart and accept things as they are.

Goy helped me to understand this connection. She and I were sitting at the house one evening when I asked her to explain the phrase *tham jai*.

"*Tham jai* . . . is a little word for *anicca*," she said. In equating the two she was essentially telling me that making the heart means to be OK with things that change; and everything changes. When Goy told me this, I asked her how making the heart, letting go, and impermanence are all connected to emotion. I wanted to know how people practice and experience emotions that were not as riled or agitated as I was used to, how they keep a "feeling" in a sensory mode from turning into an "emotion" in the robust, affective one. But Goy was confused by the way I was phrasing the question.

"What do you mean?" she asked. I was still trying to map Thai notions of feelings through a Western conception of emotion. I realized what I was doing, and I tried to think of a way instead to ask for an example of how she kept sensory feelings from turning into what I might think of as

---

16. The term *plong* that I have translated as "to lay it down" represents a colloquial way of talking about the letting go that nonattachment brings. It is sometimes combined with the word *anicca* itself when people talk about topics like sickness and death: "*Plonganicca*" refers to a feeling of disillusionment because of an awareness of impermanence. As one person I interviewed said when I asked the meaning of *anicca*, "*anicca* means *plong*, to let go."

the question :

an emotion. "OK, well give me an example of a bad mood, and tell me an example of a good mood. Tell me how they got that way," I said.

She told me this: "Well . . . let's say it's really, really hot in your room. Because it's the hot season, and after that it'll be the cool season. Let's say you get attached to that hotness, you can't stop thinking about it, that feeling of heat. You feel attached to the wish that it wasn't hot. You don't want it to be that way anymore. You don't let go, you get angry at it. And so you feel hot-hearted. That's how a bad mood comes to be." It had been only a few months since the incident when I had gotten angry at the heat, and in getting angry had inadvertently accused her of not caring. Her illustration brought this (shameful) memory to mind.

She went on, following my question about both bad and good moods: "But here's a good way to feel instead: you feel warm. You can be uncomfortable, but you can realize that it's the hot season. It's hot everywhere. So you feel calm, cool. You realize it's hot, you know that won't last, and you don't let that feeling of heat become a mood. You let go of that feeling. That's good."

4

Holding On

One afternoon about six months into fieldwork I noticed Gaew's father Paw Nui and a neighbor carrying something awkwardly across the street. When I looked closer I saw a pale old woman slung between their arms. It was Mae Mon, the matriarch of the family. Grandmother Mae Mon had raised Sen in Chiang Mai and had been the fiery center of the group for years, but now she was ninety-three years old and sick, and was not expected to live much longer.

"She's been staying upstairs at the house for the past year," Gaew said after her father disappeared across the street. "We're bringing her back to my parents' house to rest." Mae San and Paw Nui owned a second home in the field across the street from their shop, but they rarely used it, preferring to spend their time at the shophouse with their children.

A few weeks later Mae Mon passed away, and for the three days after her passing chairs were set up in the field near the house to accommodate the guests that showed up to pay their respects. A tent was set up with her coffin and a large portrait of her at the front. Inside the house monks chanted all day and night, their voices in a low harmony of Pali chants broadcast over a loudspeaker outside. Neighbors, including Goy, Mae Daeng, and me, visited every day, sitting at the back of the crowd listening with hands together in the Buddhist *wai*. Mae Daeng chatted quietly with neighbors and ate the snacks that Gaew was circulating as she walked around and greeted people. Gaew and Sen's parents were busily greeting guests and taking care of the monks. They were also overseeing the coffin and its visitors, as guests walked up and added incense to a large pot in front of the portrait to pay their respects. Young Noi was helping out his parents and Gaew where he could. As Gaew passed by where Mae Daeng and I were sitting, she pointed out the coffin to me. "That's where my grandmother is sleeping," she said, and laughed, her characteristic laugh of trying not to take something too seriously. Sen, for his part, was nowhere to be found.

[handwritten margin note: After her grandma died]

Mae Mon's death served as a kind of turning point for the family, and profoundly so for Sen. No one saw Sen at her funeral through all the events. I later learned that he had stayed in his room for the whole three days of the proceedings, drinking *lao khao*, the locally made rice whiskey that was sold at the back of market stalls in plastic bags for twenty baht (sixty-five cents) a sack. He did not see the body, listen to the monks, or share in the occasion with the others. He didn't take part in the rituals surrounding her death.

I ate dinner with Mae Daeng at our house a few weeks later and afterward walked over to say hello to Gaew and Sen, but as usual of late Sen was nowhere to be seen. Gaew was sitting at the main desk of the shop, Noi was playing a computer game at a desk behind her, and their parents were out of town, having left with a group in a van on one of their frequent Buddhist retreats in Chiang Mai. Pan was still at work. "Where's Sen?" I asked Gaew. I hadn't seen or heard from him in a few days, and was wondering where he had gone.

Noi looked up at me and then back at his computer game. The room suddenly felt tense. Moments went by as he and Gaew, with serious expressions and stilted body movements, hesitated to answer my question. I was taken aback by their strange response. "I don't know," Gaew replied; "I haven't seen him in a few days either."

"What? Where could he have gone? Is he all right?" I was confused, but she just smiled tensely. I left, but when I stopped by the shop again the next day he still wasn't there.

"Should we try to find him?" I asked Gaew again, worried, and again she said that she didn't know.

After a while, though, she said, quietly, "Julia, he's in his room. He hasn't come out of his room in three days."

Sen's Attachments

Gaew didn't want to talk about it, but I could tell she was worried about Sen. Sen's room was in the back of the house in an area apart from the rest of the family, a kind of raised shed by the river and a rice field, past the area the family used for storage. When he had been out near the front of the house, we would spend hours talking, and often continued our conversations on the phone at night, but I had never been to the back room. "It's not proper for you to visit my room," he'd said, "because I'm male and you're female." So I stayed away, worried.

When he appeared a few days later he was haggard and bleary-eyed. He tried to sit at the desk to manage the shop, but Gaew told him he should move to a more comfortable spot at the sofa. "I haven't slept in days," he told me quietly when she was out of the room, "and now I'm here, I want to work. But Gaew never lets me do anything. I don't have anything to do." It seemed at that moment that his comment about women being in charge was a complaint as much as an observation. I whispered to Gaew that he should manage the desk just to keep occupied. She hesitated, and said, almost desperately, "He can't, Julia. He's totally drunk!" I looked over at him and noticed his balance was off, and that he was moving slowly, holding on to the wall for support.

"We don't know what to do." Gaew pulled me aside as Sen retreated back to the darkness of his room, where he stayed for the rest of the day. She was nervous and concerned, her forehead creasing in worry; she really had no idea what to do. "We just started noticing it a few weeks ago at Mae Mon's funeral; he always drank, but typically it was with friends. After Mae Mon died it got worse."

Weeks later Sen told me that he didn't go to Mae Mon's funeral because he couldn't bear the thought that Mae Mon had died. Mae San had given Sen to Mae Mon to raise in Chiang Mai soon after he was born; he would visit his parents and his younger sister on school holidays, and when Gaew graduated high school in Mae Jaeng she joined her brother in the city to attend business school together at the junior college. When Sen and Gaew graduated, Mae Mon brought them back to live in Mae Jaeng, taking over the family shop, and Sen opened up a video rental place at one of the shop spaces connected to the store. During the first years back in Mae Jaeng, he told me, life was fun and easy; friends would stop by at all hours, and they would eat meals in front of the shop, drink, and watch the life of the town pass by. I recalled the time I had met him briefly during my first visit to Mae Jaeng; his shop was open, and he had happily rented me American films dubbed into Thai and watched them with me in the store. But after a while, I found out, he had started to close his shop early whenever he wanted to go out with friends, or open it late to sleep in; and after video rental became superseded by the internet, he found himself without customers and closed the business altogether. His friends still showed up at the store regularly, but over the next few years things slowly started to change. His friends were getting married or moving away, and his sister married a man he didn't like. And now his grandmother who had raised him had died. He began staying in his room more, coming out to tend the shop less regularly. When he did go out he drank, just as he drank when he was in.

I had noticed Sen was spending more and more time in his room, and after Mae Mon's funeral he seemed to disappear. At first, following Mae Mon's death, the extent of his drinking was a family secret. Gaew and her family pretended that nothing was wrong, smiling with only a hint of tension when people came by to ask after him. Gaew, Noi, their parents, and a few of their friends knew about it, though not the degree of it at first. In the beginning Sen still functioned relatively well, sitting at the desk when he wasn't drunk, disappearing every half hour to nip a bit from a stash of whiskey he had in the back of the house. He would go out with friends at night, to restaurants where he always drank more than they did but still participated in the conversations and fun, only sometimes sitting in silence and staring out into the dark street. He would often seem to retreat emotionally, usually in larger groups or in groups where he didn't know anyone.

"I don't want to leave the house at all," he told me as we were sitting at the shop, the hours blending into days and weeks and months looking out at the street. "Do you know when the last time was that I went to Chiang

Mai?" he asked another time. Almost everyone I knew in Mae Jaeng took the two-hour trip to the city often, at least once every month or two, for fun or business or both. On frequent trips to Chiang Mai with Gaew and Aung I rode in the back of pickup trucks like the others, up over the mountain and down the other side to the city, where they would change their shoes from countryside sandals to fancy city heels and their speech from the round Northern Thai dialect to the sharper Central one before heading out to stock up on supplies and hit the city's cafés and bars.

"Three months? Four months?" I guessed when Sen asked.

He looked at me. "I haven't left this town in over three years." He looked down the dusty street at the town's one main intersection, with its stop sign covered in dust and virtually useless.

"I can't accept that Mae Mon is gone," Sen told me regularly, as the weeks and then months passed by. I was continuing my interviews and getting to know Mae Jaeng more and more, visiting Chiang Mai every few weeks when I could, but Sen seemed to be standing still. "I can't accept the changes in Mae Jaeng," he told me. "Everyone's going here, going there. I just want to *stay*, for things to be the way they were."

One morning when Aung stopped by to visit Sen on a break from the market, the three of us sat looking out at the street from the shop, which on a Monday was especially busy with people coming down to the market from Karen and Hmong villages in the hills and others returning from their weekends in Chiang Mai. After a particularly loud truck passed by, Aung said casually, "Mae Jaeng shouldn't be like this."

"Yeah," Sen nodded in agreement. Unlike Aung, who had mentioned the traffic in passing, he continued to look blandly out to the street at the stream of people and vehicles. "It used to be that when you went around town," he said, "like, you turned the corner from the market or something, you could just go. But now you have to do like this"—he stretched his neck to look around right and left—"check out all the time for other cars. You can barely cross the street. Look—not even that dog there can cross! It used to be much nicer here. A long time ago the forest monks used to walk through, government people came to relax . . . the valley was famous and peaceful. Now look at it. It's changing too fast."

Sen liked to tell me about his time as a teenager in Chiang Mai. "When Gaew came to the city for high school we had a little red car we drove around in," he said. "Back then barely anyone had cars in Chiang Mai.

There was no traffic, not like now, and we could drive around easily. We would cruise around the streets, picking up friends and smoking and listening to music." Sen recounted this image of the little red car often, along with the time he and a carload of his friends drove up to Mae Hong Son for the weekend. "We would roll down the windows to smoke, stopping off to sleep in little towns on the way. I remember it rained a lot that day, and I remember looking out the window and thinking I wanted it to just stay like that forever." He spoke wistfully about the past in Chiang Mai and Mae Jaeng, smiling, but his tone changed when he contrasted it with how things were in the present, like the emotional distance he felt with his sister, who he said was too busy all the time. He couldn't let go.

"I want Mae Jaeng to be like the way it was," he told me again and again, as he looked out at people passing by on the street in front of the shop, or even at the monks who walked by through town from time to time on foot; and as we talked on the phone at night; and as he and I sat at the shop and watched his parents or sister leave for yet another trip to Chiang Mai. "Everyone wants to do things, go places . . . running to Chiang Mai, going out. . . . I want things to *stop*, to be the way they were. . . . Gaew and I used to be friends. Now she doesn't care about me, she just pays attention to her husband, and to the shop. Her personality has changed; she just thinks about money all the time." He would say these things in a kind of mumble, and then disappear into the back room and return with his breath smelling like whiskey. He still liked to sit at the shop and watch people go by, but he started to forget what day it was, or even what time of day. Everything seemed to be moving too fast for him.

Few other people talked to me about the past unless I asked them, and when they did they usually recalled it fondly but would also speak optimistically about the future. Sen discussed the past often, but when I would bring up the future he would become silent. When I sat down to conduct a formal interview with him I asked him to imagine the future in Mae Jaeng and to tell me about it.

"Fifteen years in the future?" He was silent for a moment, and then continued, "Nothing. I don't think it'll be like anything. I think I'll be dead then."

His response was even more unusual when I asked my interview question about what he thought would happen after death: "I won't know anything, I won't be anything," he said. "I won't be reborn, I won't be a ghost. It's over." This was markedly different from all the other responses I had heard in the interviews with people in Mae Jaeng, who all talked about karma in its many guises as the continuation of life of some sort.

A lot of Sen's ways of looking at things were unusual. "Usually he was really fun to be around," his high school friend Santi said when I asked about their time in Chiang Mai together. "But sometimes he would get into some mood I wouldn't recognize. You couldn't get him to let go of some thought he had at that point, no matter what."

"He's always been strange," Gaew said, chiming in on the conversation. "He didn't want to make friends with new people. He would get angry when our friends and I would go out and someone new would come and talk to us. I always knew I had a strange brother."

"I say things how they are, or I don't say anything at all," Sen told me matter-of-factly. His attitude of direct speech or silence was almost the opposite of what I heard from others, who emphasized an awareness of the interpersonal aspects of their feelings and the letting go of attachments rather than keeping them in or expressing them.

Sen and I had been talking on the phone for a while one night when I asked if he would help me with a project the next day, but he was upset about something Gaew's husband Pan had said to him. He told me, "If I can make my heart [*tham jai*] by tomorrow, I'll come out of my room. If I can't, you won't see me." I stopped by his house the following day, but he wasn't around; he wasn't able to make his heart. Sen knew about culturally valued emotional practices like *jai yen* and *tham jai*, and from what I could tell he even valued them; but he had trouble putting them into practice.

In an environment where the emotional tone of words and actions is important, and keeping others' interests in mind is valued, Sen often found himself saying nothing at all rather than breaching social norms.

He talked to me about the problems he was having with Pan. "Pan hates me," Sen said. "He should be deferential to me. He's younger than me, and he moved only three years ago into the house, but he acts like he owns the place. Do you know what he said to me yesterday? He told me I was lazy and no good, and that after my parents die he's kicking me out of the house! It's my house!" From my conversations with Pan I knew that Pan was concerned about Sen's health and was worried that Sen's drinking was hurting Gaew, who cared about her brother but didn't know what to do.

"Is there someone you can talk to about this?" I asked Sen. "Can you talk to Gaew?"

"She doesn't care," he said; "she's so busy with her work. She'd be caught in the middle and would probably defend him. She doesn't want to know about it."

"Your mom, then?"

"My mom should help me," he said at first, agreeing, "because I was in her womb for nine months. But I can't ask her; I feel too deferential [*kreng jai*] to her. It would upset her."

His problems with Pan stemmed in part from friction caused by there not being space in the home for both of them. If Sen had followed the pattern of most grown males in Mae Jaeng, he would have married out of the house a few years earlier and into the home of a wife. But Sen did not follow the pattern of the majority of other males in Mae Jaeng. Whether he liked it or not—and I sometimes got the feeling that he did not like it at all—he would never marry, and he was too attached to his family to move out to the city, even though his friends from time to time invited him to live there with them.

During the many days Sen and I spent at the front of the shop house we would often hear the sound of Chai's motorcycle, and Sen would get up from where he was sitting behind the desk to see him come in. Chai had recently bought a new Harley-Davidson and liked to rev the engine when he came near Sen's shop, "to let me know he's here," Sen said. Chai would walk in and say "Yo!" in a loud voice, pick out some laundry detergent or some other item, laugh when I (as often as not) gave him the wrong change for his purchase, glance briefly at Sen, and walk out again into the sun. Sen for his part would sit silently while Chai was there. Inevitably, after Chai left, he would get up and return a few minutes later smelling of rice whiskey. He wouldn't say anything, and we would return to looking at a magazine or start chatting about something else.

One late night after this had happened, Sen and I were talking on the phone about relationships, and he said, "Yeah, Chai is bi. We slept together last week." While Sen and Chai's relationship grew in private, in public they continued as casual friends. Chai in turn struggled with his attraction; Chai would pause at the table if he came to Sen's family house for dinner, not sure whether to sit next to Sen or not, or even whether to join the group for dinner at all. One night Chai's motorcycle pulled up to the restaurant by the river where Sen, Aung, Gaew, and I were sitting. He sat on his bike for a moment, unsure whether to join the group, but then left.

Sen would usually pay little attention to him, and, Chai told me, would even fail to return his call if something he'd said had made Sen upset. Sen would return home from staying out at night with Chai but then ignore him during the day.

Sen's childhood friend Lek stopped by for dinner at Sen and Gaew's shop another night, but on seeing that Chai was there waved from his motorbike and continued on.

"Why didn't Lek stay?" I asked Sen later, as we saw Lek heading home again from his evening out.

"It's because Chai's his boss," Sen said, "and he's *kreng jai*; he's deferring to Chai." Lek and Sen apparently had a long-standing flirtation. Lek sensed the relationship between his boss and friend, and out of respect he didn't interfere. When Chai did try to spend more time with Sen in public, Sen did nothing to encourage him, often neglecting to invite him over at all during a party or avoiding him altogether. However Chai felt, I never got close enough with him to tell.

"Chai's family is Chinese Thai," Sen said by way of explanation for why Chai wasn't more open about his relationship with Sen, suggesting that Chai's family wouldn't approve. "He wants to keep his family, and all the other good things in his life, and he's worried he'd lose that if he told them."

Sen and Chai were struggling with their attachment to each other, and to a much lesser extent a similar process was happening with Aung; she, too, had developed a crush on Chai. One unusually chilly night, as she sat with the others by the river, she turned to Chai and said, "Can I wear your coat? I'm cold." He smiled, took it off, and slyly handed it over to Sen instead, who gave a kind of smirk and put it on. Sen remembered the story warmly, but he also felt sorry for Aung, who, unaware of the nature of the relationship but probably sensing the intimacy between her two friends, had just said "Hey!" and laughed.

For almost a year Aung alternated between going out of her way to show up when plans involved Chai, and avoiding some social events specifically because he would be there. But she was able to let go of her attachment to him, and after a few months she started dating a nice Chinese-Thai man in town. The man she started seeing left to work for a year in a mine in southern China, and when I asked her if she missed him, she said "Yeah, but I talk to him on the phone sometimes . . . it is the way it is."

"It's bad to be attached to just one other person so much," Aung told me, reflecting on her feelings of wanting to text her new boyfriend all day. "It's like he's a possession; it's like I want to possess that person."

Aung struggled, but others were more successful in their attachments. Goy handled love in the same manner she handled most of her life: calmly and coolly. If anything, she became even calmer and cooler than I had first known her to be when, after I had been living in Mae Jaeng for about six months, she began a romantic relationship with a woman she knew from Bangkok. The two of them started staying at the stationery store where I had first met her; her friend opened an internet shop, and I would stop by to find the two of them listening to *dhamma* talks, talking, and making food as people stopped by the shop for supplies. Mae Daeng accepted Goy's friend as a daughter. Goy was not "out," in the sense of a public declaration of a sexual orientation,[1] but when an extra room opened up in the house, Mae Daeng did not ask why the friend continued to stay with Goy in her room. "Everyone knows," Sen had told me when I asked what people thought of the two of them. "When someone's single over thirty in this town, well, people assume," he added, looking at me significantly, though at the time I didn't catch the oblique reference to his own sexual orientation, which at that point he had not yet shared with me. Goy was calm and comfortable with it, and although she didn't make it public, it wasn't much of an issue for her. The emotional lives of Goy and Sen couldn't be explained simply by social disapproval of homosexuality; their experiences were quite different from each other, and the difference can be explained in part by contrasting attitudes: part of the reason for Sen's problem with his own sexuality was his inability to come to terms with it, as he told me, and accept it, rather than it being seen as inherently a problem.

---

1. The idea of a person with a homosexual orientation "coming out" by making his or her sexual orientation public may be a common trope in the United States, but it is a recently introduced concept in Mae Jaeng. "Coming out" suggests a kind of public authenticity and a public sincerity on the outside that matches one's true self, of being comfortable with the person that one "really is." The attitude is foreign in Mae Jaeng less because of explicit homophobia and more because such an attitude suggests an inner "self" along with an outer "self," and that the goal for personal well-being is for that inner self to be expressed. In Mae Jaeng this perspective is problematic, as the idea of a stable self is not a given. Most gay people I know there are neither "in the closet" nor out of it. Desire and romantic love, in this sense, were similar in both hetero- and homosexual relationships; it was not that people kept their feelings "in," but that they did not express them publicly with the purpose of creating a "sincere" public persona that matched a "true self."

Gaew and Pan for their part were a happily married couple. The way they expressed this was not through public verbal or physical pronouncements; they rarely touched or seemed to me like a couple at all in public. But late at night with close groups of friends they would sit together and tease each other and joke around. Their light humor was commented on, always in fun. People took their relationship seriously, but while caring about each other was a good thing, it was not the subject of serious discourse. In contrast to cultural values of the sanctity of marriage presided over by a religious figure, as in a Christian wedding, at marriage ceremonies in Mae Jaeng monks are relatively absent, especially compared with their visible presence at almost all other life passages. Romantic relationships in Mae Jaeng are seen to occur in spite of rather than because of religious teachings. Only once, when Gaew and I had gone on a trip and Pan was away on a work trip of his own, Gaew said to me quietly, laughing, "I miss my husband." Other than that she acted as if the two were simply good acquaintances.

Buddhist Engagements and Sen

The Buddha famously suggested that attachments are a part of everyone's (unenlightened) human life, and that all those who are not enlightened will be caught in those very attachments. Suffering (*dukkha*) is one of the Three Characteristics (Pali, *tilakkhaṇa*) of life, according to Buddhist teachings, and is understood to occur because of a concept of human nature in which people attach to things that they would like to be static but that nevertheless change.[2] At heart, attachments imply a desire for permanence: they imply a wish for things to stay the same (when these things are liked), and a desire for things to go away (when they are not), but because of the impermanence of things, such desire can never be met;

2. This is understood to be the case even for those who dedicate all their time to religious study, but such people are thought to be better at not becoming overly attached because of their religious training. "When my mom died I was sad," a monk told me, "but my brother and sister were really, really sad. I was sad, but I wasn't sad like them. I was sad, but not as much." Samuels, *Attracting the Heart* (2010), shows how "even" Buddhist monks whom Samuels knew in Sri Lanka must navigate affective ties with others even as they work toward the shared Buddhist ideal of nonattachment.

nothing is stable. The Buddhist soteriological goal thus is to exist in a state of detachment. This is the ideal. The practical aspect of Buddhism is the actual practice of becoming better and better at detaching. Everyone I know in Mae Jaeng agrees that Buddhism is right in teaching that attachments lead to suffering, and everyone struggles with attachments to some extent. The common recognition, then, that attachment is an ongoing difficulty ever present in life gives rise to an understanding of the foundational social necessity for the practice of, and cognitive elaboration on, letting go.

Letting go of attachments and the connection of such attachments to the idea of change and suffering are difficult concepts to tease apart and make sense of in the lives of Sen, Gaew, Goy, and the many others living in Mae Jaeng. When people ordain or reside at monasteries for meditation retreats, the following of Buddhist ideals can still be difficult and, as is the case everywhere, complicated by the problems of personal social life; but in such a separate space the religious ideals are explicit as the focus of practice. Outside of formal religious settings, the pushes and pulls of everyday life are even more pronounced, and Buddhist ideals are jumbled together with attitudes and obligations and desires of the home and market. People in Mae Jaeng act as if they have a self, for instance, even as they follow teachings that say there is no such thing as a self (as *anatta*, the third of the Three Characteristics, implies).[3] People like Sen, Gaew, Aung, Chai, and Goy create stability and happiness for themselves even as they know at another level that clinging to these things is an illusion that causes suffering. This is true for practically everyone in Mae Jaeng: over half the people I interviewed talked about the difficulties of aspiring to ideals in practice; they incorporated these ideals in different ways to create narratives about their

---

3. The Three Characteristics of impermanence (*anicca*), suffering (*dukkha*), and nonself (*anatta*) are deeply connected: as one middle-aged man in Mae Jaeng told me, using mostly colloquial Thai rather than formal Pali Buddhist terms, "Yes, I know about *anicca*. It's impermanence [*mai thieng*], uncertainty [*mai nae non*]. Our selves aren't ourselves [*mai chai tua ton*]. If we were ourselves, we wouldn't want to let go; we don't want to be old, to hurt, but we can't control that. It's nature. It's a normal thing—we're not really ourselves. We can't stop ourselves. We don't want to hurt. But we can't not hurt, because we don't have our own bodies. We don't want to get old, but we have to get old, because it's not our own selves. We don't want to die, but we'll die because it's not ourselves. We have to accept it [*yom*]; we can't forbid it." For more on nonself see Collins 1982; Buddhadasa 1989, the Abhidhamma, and the Visuddhimagga (Buddhaghosa [430 CE] 2003). See also Shweder and Bourne 1984; Markus and Kitayama 1991.

life.[4] They usually accompanied these kinds of comments about suffering and nonself with disclaimers, saying that they don't quite understand the teachings fully but that maybe they will in the future.

"I suffer even when I don't know it!" Aung told me. "Even when I'm doing well, *dukkha* is there, suffering is there." The same goes for the realization of self-lessness: "I know it's true, that there's no such thing as the self," I was told by one old woman, who went on, laughing, "but it's hard to understand— I've made good karma, so I'll understand more in my next life!"

It is within this ambiguous conceptual space that attachment and non-attachment play out in everyday life. Approaching the issue of attachment as either being attached (that is, feeling passionately about one or a small number of people and ideas and things over others) or nonattached (feeling equanimous and compassionately but disinterestedly detached from individual people and things of the world) represents the two extremes: one represents the wheel of suffering, and the other, enlightenment. It is hard—practically impossible, some might say—to be truly unattached, but nonattachment still serves as an aspiration in everyday life.[5]

At Noi's ordination months earlier, the head monks and the other novices with Noi intoned a chant used in all ordinations in the country, as their families listened:

> In various ways has moral conduct
> been rightly expounded,
> collectedness been rightly expounded,
> wisdom been rightly expounded
> by the Lord, the One-who-knows,
> the One-who-sees, the Arahant, the
> Perfect Buddha, for the subduing of intoxication,
> for the getting rid of thirst,

---

4. Life narratives were told when I asked about personalities and personal changes during interviews, and were also brought up spontaneously in casual conversations when a new circumstance or situation was incorporated into overarching personal stories. See McAdams, Josselson, and Lieblich 2006 and Cohler 1982 for more on theories of personal narratives and life-course perspectives on human development, especially in terms of the construction, memory, and coherence of the stories people tell of themselves.

5. It may be for this reason that some critics and scholars of Buddhist practice have mistakenly argued that everyday Buddhist practices in Thailand are "counterdoctrinal" or that people don't understand or even seriously follow the teaching.

for the uprooting of attachment,
for the breaking of the round (of re-birth),
for the destruction of craving,
for dispassion,
for cessation,
for the realization of Nibbàna.
Now when moral conduct is
thoroughly developed, collectedness
is of great fruit, of great advantage.[6]

The Pali chant wasn't in a language that the people listening or even the children speaking it understood, but the head monk residing over the proceedings explained it in the Northern Thai dialect that everyone knew.

A few weeks after Noi finished his time as a novice monk I asked if he remembered learning about *anicca* or nonattachment. He thought about it, shrugged, and said no, that he didn't, but his friend Pae, who was sitting next to him and had ordained too, elbowed him and said, "Yeah, remember? *Anicca, dukkha, anatta* ... let go." Noi nodded noncommittally in response, and the two of them turned their attention back to their computer game. For them it was a passing thought, and for me it was a reminder that the iterations of learning are long term rather than immediate, and that everyone learns and remembers lessons differently.

Sen was familiar with Buddhist teachings, but for the most part he did not practice them. At Noi's ordination, dozens of relatives had been there, but when I asked Gaew where Sen was, she said, "He's at home, sleeping. He doesn't come to things like this."

"You know, Sen has never ordained," Mae San told me one day while she and Gaew and I were driving in the truck through the mountains on the way to Chiang Mai. She seemed disappointed when she said this, as if it was an explanation of some sort, but she spoke matter-of-factly, and I stayed quiet. I was surprised to hear that. Virtually all males in Mae Jaeng, as in the rest of Thailand, ordain at some point in their life. "Sen doesn't

---

6. This chant is called the Anusàsana (the admonishment for Bhikkhus), in the "Ordination Procedure [Upasampadàvidhā] and the Preliminary Duties of a New Bhikkhu," compiled by HRH Supreme Patriarch Somdet Phra Mahà Samaōa Chao Krom Phrayà Vajiraàōavarorasa Mahàmakuñaràjavidyàlaya, trans. Mr. Siri Buddhasukh and Phra Khantipàlo, King Mahà Makuta's Academy, Bangkok, 2516/1973.

know what's going on,"[7] she finished. Sen was already thirty-two years old, but other than an old Burmese man covered in tattoos whom I had met at the edge of town, he was the only one I knew who had never ordained.

"I can't go there," Sen said when I asked him later why he never went to the wat, even to make merit. I had gone with Gaew to the wat on dozens of occasions, or had seen her there when I went with Mae Daeng, but even at Noi's ordination, when so many extended family members were present, he hadn't entered the grounds: "You can't go to the wat," he told me by way of explanation, "if you've been drinking."

I had seen Goy encounter a drunk man lying in the monastery grounds in the countryside once; even though he was probably twice her age and in that sense her superior, Goy had spoken to him harshly: "What are you doing drunk at the wat!" she had said to him. "You can't do that—get out of here!" I had been surprised at her tone talking to someone older than she was, when usually she was so respectful, but I also remembered the Buddhist precept against intoxication. At the many wat festivals in town there was a prodigious amount of drinking, but it always took place outside the monastery grounds themselves. Sen, always drunk now, felt he couldn't go into the wat grounds at all. But his drinking was just a part of his reasoning. He was "bored" with religious life, he told me, and didn't feel like he was or wanted to be a part of it.[8]

Sen continued: "I respect the Buddha. But the monks, we don't know who they are, what they do. I don't want to bow down to them, I don't know them. I don't like those ritual things." The dislike of ritual extended to his home, too. "I used to chant before I went to sleep," he told me, "but then I just stopped." Others I knew preferred some ritual practices over others also, but Sen seemed to have a blanket antagonism against religious

---

7. The phrase she used, *mai ruu ruang*, connotes something stronger and more general than just "doesn't know what's going on." Literally it translates as "doesn't know the story" and relates to someone who is ignorant or out of step with what is happening around him.

8. See Cassaniti 2015a for a discussion of "boredom" in Thai religious life, drawing from an analysis by Dumm (1999). In addition to avoiding the monastery because he was drinking, or bored, Sen also may have hesitated to engage with the ritual options around him because of his sexuality. Part of the ordination process is to affirm that one is a "real man," which some homosexual males have felt has kept them from the monkhood. Michael Chladek (forthcoming) discusses some of the nuances of this last possibility in his study of homosexuality and the monkhood in Northern Thailand.

practice. He knew a lot about Buddhist philosophy, and I could tell that he respected it, but socially it didn't seem like an option to him.

A lot of the problems that Sen had were practical and specific to him and to his particular situation in life: his difficulty with his brother-in-law was a problem in a place where only married sons left the parents' home; his homosexuality was a problem in a place that he felt didn't socially accept it; his upbringing by his grandmother was a problem; and an appreciation for traditional small-town culture was a problem in a place of rapidly increasing modernization and friends who were moving on. These were all individual problems that together propelled the larger problem, but the issue of not being able to let go was understood to undergird all of them. The drinking itself was a symptom as much as a cause of his increasing unhappiness.

I watched the way Gaew laughed off her cares, neither fully expressing them nor keeping them in, allowing them instead to diffuse, because she knew that holding on to them would bring her unhappiness. I watched the way Mae Daeng, Goy, Aung, Chai, and others did so too. But Sen didn't do this. "I want to say things, but I can't," he told me. He wanted to tell people he cared about them, to ask his mom for help with his problems with Pan, to ask his sister to be his friend again, to either be with Chai as a couple or else not feel so attached to him. He wanted things to be the way they were in the past, but he found that he couldn't express his feelings. He couldn't, somehow, let his feelings go. It seemed that sometimes Sen's emotion patterns were less an issue of right or wrong, of universally healthy or not healthy, but more an issue of a mismatch with the patterns of people in his immediate social surroundings. He knew he shouldn't get attached, but he did, and this, he said, was why he drank. And it wasn't specifically that he was gay—lots of his friends were gay—or because of other particular situations like his grandmother's death or his brother-in-law's encroachment on his home. It was the attachment he felt, to one particular friend, to his grandmother, to his sister in the past, and to the past in general—these were the problems that lay beneath the practical ones in front of him.

Attachment and Impermanence in Ban Ko Tao

I sat at Duansri's shop in Ban Ko Tao glumly one afternoon, thinking about Sen. As Duansri and I shucked tamarinds, reaching over periodically to put coins that customers handed us for their purchases into the wicker basket of money, we talked about Sen's problems. I was feeling angry at Sen's parents for not doing more, and even felt angry at the model of emotionality I was seeing around me that seemed to usually work for people but that I felt was somehow failing Sen. I was even angry at myself for not being able to be the distant observing anthropologist I had read about before my fieldwork, who wrote things down that people said and did and took part in activities but kept an "objective" distance from them. My friends had become personal friends and not just subjects, and I wasn't sure what to do about it. Duansri knew Sen and his family from when Sen's father had taught school years before at the Karen village farther up the hill, and was surprised when I told her about Sen's problems with alcohol.

"Why don't they do something!" she asked, meaning Sen's parents. "They should yell at him, get mad at him. Tell him to stop. Not just do nothing. I would do that. That's what people do here." She ended her comments with, "Sometimes you have to get angry."

I agreed with her, but I knew that she and I were both drawing in our own ways from our own perspectives on emotion and attachment and action, and that it wasn't the way things worked in Mae Jaeng. In their own way Sen's parents weren't doing nothing; as his mother reminded me when I talked to her about Sen, she felt they needed to wait and accept what was happening, that they were trying to create change through acceptance. It just seemed like nothing to Duansri. I had already noticed that in Ban Ko Tao, robust emotionality and talk about problems were more commonly emphasized, and the emphasis was made even more evident when the subject of Sen and his drinking came up.

"We'll pray to God for him," the pastor Jerapong told me when the news of Sen's problems reached him.

The idea of supposed efficacy from talking with divinity, with other people, and even with professional mental health workers was much more common in the Christian community than what I was used to in Mae Jaeng. I was visiting friends at the hospital in Mae Jaeng a few weeks after talking to Duansri about Sen when I ran into Surree, a Karen woman I knew from Ban Ko Tao. Surree was an intelligent, gregarious woman who loved to read and at twenty-two had just gotten married.

"What are you doing here?" I asked her, not having previously seen her outside her village.

"I think there's something wrong with me," she replied, and she told me about it as we sat together in the waiting room waiting for the doctor to call her name. "There's something wrong with my mind," she said; "I'm unsatisfied with my life; everyone in Ban Ko Tao goes out to the rice fields in the daytime and comes home and cooks and watches TV. That's all they do. They're happy with it, but I'm not. So I come here to talk to a psychologist about my problems." I was surprised by her comfort in talking about her problems, and even more surprised that there was a psychologist to talk with, because I had heard from both Ban and Jiew, two of Sen's friends who worked in the hospital in Mae Jaeng, that there wasn't anyone like that. I was also surprised at how different Surree's way of thinking was from what I was used to in Thai Buddhist discussions of mental health in Mae Jaeng: Surree described her troubles and laid out the solution, which was to talk to a psychologist. No one in Sen's family or circle of friends had heard of or sought out this kind of care. On hearing her name called out over the loudspeaker, Surree got up and headed into the doctor's room, and I walked over to the pharmacy counter to say hi to Ban. When I next saw Surree, back in Ban Ko Tao, she didn't elaborate on her visit, but she seemed cheerful, and seemed to be doing well.

Not only was expressive discussion more common in Ban Ko Tao than in Mae Jaeng, but I noticed that practices of letting go that were so common in Mae Jaeng were relatively absent in Ban Ko Tao. When I asked people in the Karen village in interviews how they felt when money and other things were lost or stolen, compared with those in Mae Jaeng they told me more often that they felt angry, or sad, or that they went to the district office to track the item down. In Mae Jaeng people consistently told me that they didn't feel very angry or sad in the face of loss, and instead told me about karma (of their own and of any thieves involved), and feelings of letting go and making the heart.[9]

In Mae Jaeng people had told me that when someone they knew was in the hospital from an accident or was very sick or had passed away, they would get a call from Moh Bom, the head doctor, who would tell them to *tham jai*, to make the heart and try to accept what he was about to tell them. In Ban

---

9. In my formal interviews I found significant differences in attitudes toward monetary and other material loss in the Buddhist and Christian communities. While Christians in Ban Ko Tao were more likely to feel upset at loss and to take measures to reclaim it, Buddhists in Mae Jaeng were more likely to feel *ploy* or OK about this loss. Because I found it hard to believe that people felt OK about monetary and material loss I did a small follow-up study with forty people a year later and got similar results.

Ko Tao no one mentioned Moh Bom offering this advice, even though he, as the region's main medical doctor, did talk with them about illness and loss in their families. This difference in reported memory was either because Moh Bom knew that the idea of making the heart was not a shared component of the cultural and religious landscape in Ban Ko Tao (which would require a level of explicit reflection I wasn't sure he had), or because he did offer the same advice to people in Ban Ko Tao that he did in Mae Jaeng, but the people in Ban Ko Tao did not recall him saying it. Both possibilities would suggest that *tham jai* is a less culturally elaborated orientation in Ban Ko Tao than in Mae Jaeng. When I asked Moh Bom about the two patterns of recollections of him in the two communities, he raised his eyebrows and told me that he didn't purposely act differently in helping people in the two communities, but he nodded to both possibilities when I suggested them.

Thai-language speakers in the Karen, Christian community know and use the phrase *tham jai*, and they do not think of it as an overly Buddhist term that they might want to avoid because of their Christian beliefs (unlike words such as *kam*, or karma, which were seen as clearly Buddhist and generally avoided), but *tham jai* is not a common emotional practice to anywhere near the extent it is in the Buddhist community.

Part of why letting go seemed to make sense for people in Mae Jaeng was an awareness of change; suffering results from attaching to things. Everything changes, Buddhist religious logic suggested, and it is because of the ubiquity of change that letting go is the healthy thing to do, so I was curious if a similar concept of change was present in the Karen communities. People talked about change in colloquial terms there, but when I asked directly, only a third of those I interviewed in Ban Ko Tao knew of the word *anicca*. This could have been because even as most people in Ban Ko Tao spoke Thai, *anicca* is a technical and, officially, a Pali word explicitly linked to Buddhism: to make sure the difference wasn't one of language rather than concept I asked those who did say they knew the term *anicca* to tell me a Karen gloss. The phrase I was told in response was *tah guh law guh law*, which was then back-translated by others into Thai as *mai mii prayot*. In English *mai mii prayot* means roughly "useless," or "without benefit." When I asked people in Ban Ko Tao for concrete examples of *tah guh law guh law*, three gave me the same political one to illustrate: the then prime minister, Thaksin, had made promises that were *tah guh law guh law*, they said—useless and without benefit.

"When Thaksin was campaigning to be prime minister," one man proclaimed, "he said if elected he would give every village a buffalo. But then when he was elected he just gave each village the sperm of a buffalo, which is different. His promise was *tah guh law guh law*: useless."

The connections between the phrase *tah guh law guh law* and *anicca* are tenuous. When I asked if there was any religious meaning to *tah guh law guh law*, or to Thai colloquial terms regarding change that had been related to me in Mae Jaeng as similar to *anicca*, I was told by most people that there wasn't. But three people told me that there was, and all three pointed to the same section of the Christian Bible to explain the connection: the Old Testament's book of Ecclesiastes.

I found the passage they referred me to in a Thai-Karen-English Bible at Chiang Mai's Payap University Library; in English it read: "Vanity of vanities, says the Teacher, vanity of vanities! All is vanity. . . . What has been is what will be, and what has been done is what will be done; there is nothing new under the sun." The term "vanity" was translated from the Hebrew *hevel*: "vapor." In some English Bibles the term that usually reads "vanity" is translated instead as "useless," "meaningless," "absurdity," "frustration," or "futility."[10] In Thai the passage reads "Anicca! Anicca!" In Karen it reads "tah guh law guh law."

Anicca, vanity, and *tah guh law guh law* are translated as glosses of each other, but the impermanence in the Thai Pali word *anicca* seemed to me only slightly connected to the English "vanity," or to the lack of benefit suggested in the Karen phrase *tah guh law guh law*. And with its citation in a part of the Bible with which few in Ban Ko Tao are familiar (as the New Testament is used much more so than the Old), and which the Israeli Buddhist studies scholar Michal Pagis once told me is the most "Buddhist" part of the Bible, it seemed that neither *anicca* nor *tah guh law guh law* played a very central role in the religious life of the community, nor carried with it the same kind of religiously elaborated connotations. I later saw an English-Karen-Thai Bible that the pastor's wife Sada had at the back of a bookshelf at her house, and read in it a preface to Ecclesiastes. In English it read:

> The book of Ecclesiastes contains the thoughts of "the Philosopher," a man who reflected deeply on how short and contradictory human life is, with

---

10. New Living Bible translation 1996, Tyndale Charitable Trust; New King James Version 1982, Thomas Nelson.

its mysterious injustices and frustrations, and concluded that "life is use-less." He could not understand the ways of God, who controls human destiny—yet, in spite of this, he advised people to work hard, and to enjoy the gifts of God as much and as long as they could. Many of the Philoso-pher's thoughts appear negative and even depressing. But the fact that this book is in the Bible shows that Biblical faith is broad enough to take into account such pessimism and doubt. Many have taken comfort in seeing themselves in the mirror of Ecclesiastes and have discovered that the same Bible which reflects these thoughts also offers the hope in God that gives life its greater meaning. (Thai Holy Bible, 1971)

This fairly lengthy discussion of what amounts to a fairly insignifi-cant part of religious life in the Karen community may seem relatively insignificant to the larger issues of impermanence, emotion, and attach-ment in the everyday psychology of people in Mae Jaeng, but its relative insignificance in Ban Ko Tao is part of a larger point: impermanence as a relatively absent concept in the Karen Christian community highlights its relative importance in the Buddhist community. "The differences among languages are those of 'emphasis,'" Benjamin Whorf has said, "or of rela-tive ease in making some distinction which might be of use in certain cir-cumstances" (Whorf 1956, 147–48); this is true for attitudes reflected in the different terms and relative lack of prominence for talk about change in Ban Ko Tao compared to Mae Jaeng. The differences do not reflect dif-ferences of fundamental potentials; instead they show tendencies in how people demarcate ideas and make distinctions about experience.

I had wanted to see a coherent cultural logic in Ban Ko Tao that con-nected, say, an emphasis on discourse and robust emotions to a religious sense of permanence, or at least to the absence of an emphasis on imper-manence, in order to make a neat parallel comparative argument to the one unfolding in Mae Jaeng. But while the emphasis of the soul living on or the importance of speaking to Jesus to solve problems that I heard about in church may relate to the relatively more robust discursive emotionality I felt around me in Ban Ko Tao, they also may not. In the end I felt able to conclude only that some aspects of emotional religious life in Mae Jaeng are less relevant to everyday experience in Ban Ko Tao, and that this points to a cultural specificity of emotion and change in the Buddhist community. Comparative cases may be useful as foils in this sense, drawing attention to a normative practice by their differences, but because the categorical terms being used are constructed through attention to the main group, they are never equal in revealing two different sets of practices. In the end the main success of paying attention to my own practices, and those of other foreigners and of friends in Ban Ko Tao, was to show by way of contrast how much letting go is emphasized in Mae Jaeng.

Alcohol and the Escalation of Sen's Problems

Months were passing by, and I started to notice changes unfolding in people who had at first seemed to be relatively static personalities. I continued eating meals with Mae Daeng and Goy when I was home, and interviewing with Ari on alternate weekdays and transcribing and translating the results on the other days in a back office at his school, but I found myself spending more and more time at Sen and Gaew's house with their family and friends. In interviews, people's narratives about experiences and feelings felt real and poignant, but they also had a retrospective and packaged quality to them even if they were being packaged for the first time in the telling. With Goy, Mae Daeng, Gaew, Sen, and others I was getting to know well, I could see events happen in front of me, and could see larger situations build and unfold and reveal more subtle meanings than snapshot pictures in surveys or interview questions were able to capture.

Sen's problems were important to those around him, but I was reminded that knowing someone over time sometimes can blind one to situations that are more apparent when time doesn't blend into them. When an American friend stopped in to visit from her field site on a neighboring mountain and saw Sen for the first time in months, she took me aside after the three of us shared a meal and told me how truly awful Sen looked: "His skin is yellow, and his hands were shaking when we were talking." He had thrown uncooked rice into our dishes instead of salt by accident, and was sweating as he presented them to us.

A childhood friend of Sen who had come to visit also immediately noticed the problem. He had returned home one day from Sydney, Australia, where he had gone to live. Chang came into the shop where Sen was sitting, showing me pictures of his family trip years ago to Singapore. Chang called out "Hey!" loudly and welcomingly to Sen, but almost immediately switched tones: "Hey, what's wrong? Is that whiskey in this glass?" He could smell Sen's breath. "Hey, it's only 1 p.m.!" Chang chatted for a minute and then left the shop, leaving Sen gazing after him. "I really want to see him," Sen said to me quietly. "I want to talk to him, to go after him. But I can't."

Sen as a contrastive case was different from my own case or that of people in Ban Ko Tao; Sen was inscribed within, rather than apart from, the larger cultural orientations of his community, and his problems were understood within them.

Gaew and Sen's parents were concerned about him, but they figured the problem was one that would sort itself out, and that letting it do so was the best action to take. I felt angry at them—why didn't they do more? They had gotten involved in their formal religious practices of *yo reh*, the Japanese-Thai sect they followed. Their way of dealing with this situation was, among other things, to wear amulets of the Buddha and hold up their hands in *wai* in front of Sen to use the interpersonal exchange as a conduit of the power of the Buddha in order to transfer positive energy to him. They were away for days or more at a time at meetings or retreats in Chiang Mai, and it seemed to me in my worries and cultural conflicts that they could have done more to help him. My struggle was a cultural one, though, and I knew it reflected ideas different from theirs about what was best to do.

Pan, Gaew's husband, who did not get along with Sen, did not try to help; Noi was too young to do much; if Sen had been in a relationship with a woman, or if his relationship with Chai was socially recognized, that close other person might have advocated for him in terms of getting him help, but this wasn't the case. I was a close friend, but as a foreigner I felt that I didn't know enough or carry enough social weight to make a change. Gaew alone felt responsible for helping Sen, and she didn't know what to do.

"I tell him, 'You don't need to drink,' you know," Gaew said to me one day at the store while Sen lay passed out in a deep sleep on a mat, "and I tell him we should go see a doctor, but he doesn't listen to me."

"I told him to stop drinking," Chai told me, too, during one of our rare long conversations. Chai and I had gone swimming together one day, and he said, "Sen will call me and talk incoherently in the middle of the night, and I try to tell him to stop drinking, but if I tell him to stop too much he gets mad at me and doesn't call me, which doesn't help either."

He looked lost, unsure of how to do more, and swam off to continue his laps in the pool.

When I talked to Sen about his drinking he became silent, just as he would when Chai or anyone else talked to him about it, and would stare off into the distance blankly or with a slight scowl on his face. "It helps me just be," he told me on the rare times I did get him to talk about it. "I feel too much. The drinking helps me not feel so much, to not think too much, just be." He used the words *chuey chuey* to describe this emotional comportment he wanted to feel. *Chuey chuey* can have, depending on the context, both positive and negative connotations in Thai; it can reflect an unriled, even "equanimous" demeanor on one hand, but it can also reflect an attitude of uncaring lack of interest not contained in the more general socially valued concept of *jai yen*.

In Mae Jaeng, it is rare to attend a social event in which alcohol is not present. Goy didn't drink, because of the Chinese-Thai system of vegetarianism she followed,[11] and neither did Mae Daeng; but at any celebration, Gaew's family, like others in the neighborhood, almost always included beer and a bottle of Johnnie Walker Black, or one of the cheaper alternatives of Somsang or Mekong. Drinking is a family social practice in Mae Jaeng; husbands and wives, grown children and their parents, drank together, especially the men.[12] The prevalence of alcohol around him no doubt lured Sen in. "I remember drinking back as early as fifteen years old," he told me. "I would go out with friends in Chiang Mai, and we would all drink." On another occasion when I brought up his addiction,

---

11. In Thailand, vegetarianism is considered a good Buddhist practice and is understood to reflect one of the Five Precepts of Buddhism (to refrain from killing), but the majority of monks in Thailand do eat meat, saying that it is only proper and right to take the food offered to them as beggars. There are two main systems of practice available for those who do not eat meat. One is called *mangsawirat*, which comes from the Santi Asoke line of Thai Buddhism, in which practitioners go barefoot and eat eggs and dairy but not meat. The other, which Goy follows, is called *jey*, which comes from Chinese Buddhist influences (sometimes associated with the cult of *Avalokiteshvara*-originated Guan Im), and practitioners refrain from meat, eggs, dairy, and a range of other products thought to unhealthily "heat" up the body, including alcohol, garlic, and ice.

12. Alcoholism is a growing, widespread problem in Thailand. In recent years it has become more visible as a social issue, with tighter government restrictions on the sale of alcohol (including earlier bar closings and restricted times of the day for alcohol sales in stores) and more public-awareness campaigns (including graphic *Mao Mai Khap*—don't drink and drive—billboards at many of the country's intersections). But thousands of people develop an addiction to alcohol every year anyway. As in Sen's case, the problem is often kept a secret by family members and friends. I

Sen told me, "Everyone drinks when they socialize. If I didn't drink it would be odd, it wouldn't be accepted. I have to drink." Sen didn't think his way of doing things, in terms of his drinking, his tendency to speak directly (an uncommon speaking style in Mae Jaeng), or being silent in social contexts in which discussion was more normal, was right or good, but he couldn't seem to change it and let things go. He wanted time to stop for him, and it almost did; his eyes were so yellow from jaundice by this point that he couldn't even read the clock on the wall if he'd wanted to.

I had heard that a predisposition toward alcoholism might be rooted in one's genetic line, so I asked Gaew what she knew about their family history of drinking. When I was first getting to know him, Sen had told me that when he was young his father used to drink a lot: "He used to drink and I didn't like it, so I would hide beer from him and tell him to stop. Then he found *yo reh*, the Buddhist thing, and he quit. Now he'll drink a little bit sometimes, but not much." When I asked Gaew about a family history of drinking, she hesitated and then said, "Yeah, my dad drank a lot. And my grandfather would drink a lot too. He died in his early seventies, probably from drinking. But Sen's still young—he doesn't think it's a big issue. And he doesn't want to see a doctor, or go to Chiang Mai. But you can see his eyes are yellow, his skin is yellow, he can't see well or even walk well. It's a real problem for him."

His family and friends sometimes used the English word "alcoholism" when they referred to his problem (*"pen rok alcoholism,"* they would say, using the English term that was starting to infiltrate the Thai language— "he has the disease of alcoholism"). But more often and more colloquially they would say that he was *"dtit lao"*—addicted to alcohol. "To be addicted" and "to be attached" are the same in Thai: *"dtit." Phu dtit ya* or *dtit ya sep dtit* means a person who is addicted to drugs; if he stops his attachment/addiction, it is said he has *yut dtit*. "Whatever will happen will happen," a woman linked the two in an interview; *"ploy*, let go. We shouldn't stick to something: *mai yut dtit."*

---

once saw, at a gallery show at the Chiang Mai University Art Museum, a vivid description of the issue by a student, who had been prompted by her professor to depict it for an exhibition on family secrets: "My brother lives in the back of our house," she wrote. "He never goes out. People think he's moved to a different town. No one knows he's there, drinking." My housemate in Chiang Mai told me a similar story about his own brother. For more on alcohol use and its trends in relation to health, gender, and religion in the country see Thamarangsi 2013; Thavorncharoensap et al. 2010; Assanangkornchai, Conigrave, and Saunders 2002; Assanangkornchai et al. 2010.

Usually Sen drank his plastic-sandwich-bag-size sacks of the cheap local rice whiskey called *lao khao*, or he drank the cheap bottles of national whiskey that his family sold behind the counter at their shop, or took some change from the drawer to go to the liquor stands to get something to bring home. No one knew what to do. Gaew and I and almost all his friends stopped drinking either in front of him or altogether, and when we did drink we wouldn't invite him to join us; but not inviting him out and not drinking with him seemed to alienate and isolate him even more. He soon stopped leaving the house at all, and when he did he would drink until he looked out around him with a stony, heavy silence. When he managed to come out of his room he could barely walk straight.

Sen drank more than anyone I had ever met, but he never got angry while drinking, which seemed unusual, given the cultural stereotype I was used to of the angry alcoholic.[13] He was initially either in a pleasant mood or sullen and silent. However, as time took its toll, he would often just seem to be in a kind of blurry haze. His mom, while sitting with Sen and me at the shop one afternoon, said quietly and firmly to him at one point, "Sen, Julia and I will take you to Chiang Mai tomorrow to see the doctor about your health. You have to go. I'm your mother, and you have to do what I say." But he refused. That was the only time I heard her speaking directly to him about the problem; instead she and Paw Nui spent hours doing *yo reh* on him, sitting upright silently with a hand facing him, drawing energy, they told me, from the Buddha amulet they each wore around their necks, while Sen lay on the couch. But as far as I could tell, no one around him asked him about his personal problems.

I wondered if talking about his feelings with a professional might help. "What about a psychologist, a psychiatrist, someone he could talk to?" I asked Chai, thinking of my encounter with Surree from Ban Ko Tao.

"We don't have someone like that around here. This is a tiny town. I think there's a psychiatrist at the hospital in Chiang Mai," he said. "But anyway, it's not the way people do things here. It's not how we take care of problems."

---

13. An article in the *New Yorker* (Gladwell 2010) discusses a group of people in South America with particular patterns of drunken behavior that are quite different from those of Americans. The article argues that the social behaviors associated with drunkenness are culturally as well as biologically shaped.

During the few times Sen would appear from the back room, blinking in the sun as he shuffled in nervous fits and starts to the desk to sit down, Gaew would put a hand on his shoulder and shoo him away, saying "It's OK," quietly and kindly, "you don't have to sit here. We've got it covered." Sen would walk away and sit down on the mat in front of the store instead, falling into what he described to me in a moment of coherence as a deep, dreamless sleep.

"We don't want him managing the shop desk anymore," Gaew told me when I asked about it later. "He's blurry. He won't count the change right. He'll scare the people coming into the store. He'll take money from the drawer to go buy alcohol. And the whiskey we keep behind the desk for sale, he'll take that too, I've seen him."

"Maybe you should stop selling alcohol in your shop," I suggested to her. "Having it around makes it easier for him to get it, and to see other people getting it probably makes it feel more OK to him when he drinks."

"We can't stop selling it," she said. "People come in here to buy whiskey and beer. If I stopped selling it we would go out of business."

Almost all of Sen's friends other than Aung worked at the small Mae Jaeng hospital just a few hundred meters from his house, and they all knew he needed his blood tested for health problems, and needed a doctor to help him to stop drinking.

"But I know the people there," Sen told me in private when I suggested he visit the hospital. "I'm scared of needles. They would take my blood. It would hurt. People would see me. Nothing's wrong. I'm not going there."

Sen never admitted his drinking was a problem. "He doesn't accept it," his family and friends repeated to each other. They used the expressions *"yom rap"* (to pick up or acknowledge a situation) and *"tham jai"* when they said this. "He doesn't *yom*: he doesn't accept."

One night, long after the problem had become obvious to those around him, I stopped by one of Mae Jaeng's restaurants and found the hospital's head doctor, Moh Bom, having dinner along with Jiew, Bank (a nurse), and Ban—all of them except the doctor Sen's friends since childhood. They were eating fish and drinking whiskey by the river. I sat down with them, and we talked about Mae Jaeng.

"People here in Mae Jaeng care about each other more than in the United States," Jiew told me, half joking around. "Like, I heard that in America kids have to leave their parents' homes when they grow up. Here we all live with our parents even though we're adults. Because we watch out for each other." I disagreed, and we traded barbs about each other's cultural backgrounds, but after generalizing, the conversation took a more serious and personal note.

Moh Bom said, "Julia, we're worried about Sen." The others nodded in agreement. Jiew spoke strongly to me, the others chiming in with their support. They implored me to help him, in a kind of direct diatribe that may have been helped by their own present slight drunkenness. "What are you going to do, Julia?" Jiew said. "You have to help, it's your obligation."

Moh Bom said, "Mae San came and talked to me a few days ago. She said Sen will come out of his room to talk to you and then go back in, and that's it. He won't talk to or come out for anyone else." Jiew and the others and I brainstormed. Even though Chai had been clear that there were no Western psychiatric services in Mae Jaeng, Jiew, who was an aide at the hospital, said when I prompted toward the topic, "I know a nurse at the hospital who sometimes works as a psychiatrist." But she was away, and he didn't know when she would be back. They argued more adamantly as the conversation progressed, going back and forth about what to do.

Jiew said he knew what was really wrong with Sen: "The problem is that he's stuck in the past. He can't let go of it. Back then we were all friends, and would go out all the time. He and I were best friends. We'd stay over together every night and hang out all the time. But that was ten years ago!" Jiew laughed, and the others nodded. "Now we have families, we've moved on, grown. Sen doesn't really have any friends—you and Aung are his only friends."

"He has other friends," I said. Bank, who shared a house with Chai at the back of Mae Jaeng's hospital grounds, replied quietly, "He has Chai." I nodded in agreement, but added, "He has other friends too."

"He has drinking friends," Jiew went on, "but not people he can really talk to, like us. His parents are stressed out. But here in Mae Jaeng, it's not our culture to talk directly. We can't talk to his parents about it. It's not our place. His parents can't talk to him about it . . . his friends can't do it . . . this is a real life situation. What are you going to do, Julia?"

I laughed (as I was taught was an appropriate response to even stressful situations), and talked with them about strategies that might work, but I was also angry at them for putting so much pressure on me. It seemed that if Sen's friends cared about him, they would do something themselves.

But I also knew that they *were* doing something; they were going out of their own comfort zone to talk to me. They asked me to do something, in part because they felt uncomfortable breaking with social patterns, and assumed it wouldn't bother me as much to cause an infraction in what they might have considered a family issue. It was in this way that they felt they could help. But I didn't know what to do. I didn't feel that it was my place to intervene. I was an outsider, and an anthropologist who had been taught to observe and participate but not become too involved. Instead, in the weeks that followed, I watched and worried and talked to Sen about his drinking when I could, but I wasn't sure how to do more. I found phone numbers for rehabilitation centers in Chiang Mai and gave them to Gaew, but she had already looked into the option and dismissed it as impractical.

"I went and talked to the head doctor at Rongban Suan Prung when I was in Chiang Mai last week," she said, referring to Northern Thailand's regional psychiatric and addiction hospital, "and he said Sen could come in any time. But Sen won't do it." I looked up numbers for Alcoholics Anonymous in Chiang Mai, but with its emphasis on talk and Christian ideological undertones, I wasn't surprised to find that although there were a few Thai members, most of those using the program there were expatriates from Australia, Europe, and the United States. I had heard of a Thai monastery called Wat Tham Krabok in Central Thailand that dealt with issues of addition, but it was too far away for Sen, and his unwillingness to participate in formal Buddhist activities made it a less than ideal option.

Sen slowly went from spending afternoons to days to weeks and then months in his room. Gaew and Mae San and Paw Nui alternated between making him food to put by his door so he would have something to eat and at other times deciding not to, hoping he would come out to cook for himself. They didn't stop caring about him or stop trying to find ways to persuade him to change or get help, but other than the few times that Mae San quietly told him to see a doctor, they didn't speak to him about his problem or "lose their tempers" or yell at him to stop. They worked to remain calm and cool, and accept what was happening. But Sen was getting worse.

Part III

KARMA

5

Cause and Effect

"Let's say you did something bad, how would you feel?" Gaew asked rhetorically one day, after I asked her to explain karma to me. When I didn't reply, she went on: "You would feel bad. And that bad feeling would affect you. That's all, that's karma." She continued to elaborate, describing a local religious theory of moral causation. If you have a *sabai jai*," she said, "if you have a good, comfortable heart, then good things will happen to you. People whose hearts are good, calm, and happy are more likely to have good things happen to them." She went on: "Bad things can happen to them, too, just like bad things happen to people without a lot of good karma, but there's a difference. People with good hearts can *ploy*, they can let go, so they'll feel OK. They'll change their life and adapt, so their life will become good again."

Karma might appear to be a straightforward idea: as its English glosses suggest, "You get what you deserve," or "What goes around comes around." In Thai, karma is usually discussed fairly straightforwardly, too: "*Tham dii dai dii, tham chua dai chua*," people will say, shrugging offhandedly at its self-evident nature: "Do good and meet with good, do bad and meet with bad," echoing a phrase found in speech and school textbooks throughout the country.

But the way karma is understood to work is complicated.[1] Unlike a general sense of things changing that people in all times and places may feel, the felt reality of karma is not typically as graspable for people who have not grown up with it. As a description of moral causation, karma is about actions that carry with them the seeds of their effects. It helps to explain suffering and health, and even as its mechanisms are often downplayed in a modernized Buddhist philosophy, it is central to constructions of action and reaction in Mae Jaeng.

To nineteenth-century rationalist, modernist, and "scientific" British and Thai reinterpreters of Buddhist thought, karma came to be associated with an imagined pre-Buddhist past, a "survival" in the anthropologist Edward Tylor's sense of a cultural leftover, connected more with Hinduism than a "real" or "authentic" Buddhism. Karma is not a prominently addressed concept in English-language Buddhist scholarship, beyond a "superstitious" belief rooted in ritual. But in Mae Jaeng, karma is considered to be a cosmological entity that is obvious, true, and everywhere. Karma is real for people in Mae Jaeng, especially insofar as that an adherence to it produces effects. "Karma is like gravity," I was told more than once: "It just is."

What karma is and how it works is thought to be unambiguous, like gravity, but to an (unenlightened) mind that can't see the causes and effects of past actions, it is thought to be vague and mysterious. This is true for one's own karma, and is especially true for events that happen to others. People I knew in Mae Jaeng invoked karma to explain why things had happened to someone (phrased as "it's their karma"). When I asked people

---

1. Karma is used to sum up not just the Thai Buddhist theory of karma but often also the whole of the Buddha's teaching with it. Over forty people I interviewed quoted the phrase *tham dii dai dii, tham chua dai chua* directly in some version, and virtually everyone mentioned karma in some form during the course of explaining why some thing or other had occurred. For more on karma see Doniger O'Flaherty's (1980) analysis of karma in religious texts from South and Southeast Asia; Keyes and Daniel (1983) for ethnographic accounts of karma in practice in Theravada Buddhist contexts; and Buddhadasa Bhikkhu (2009) for a modernist take on Thai Buddhist conceptualizations of karma. Also see Cassaniti (2012, 2014a) and Carlisle (2012) for more on karma and its connections to emotion, cosmology, and belief in Thailand.

in my interviews why they thought the Andaman tsunami had occurred, a third of the people I talked with said it was due to karma of some kind, though one monk told me, "I can't answer that. It's the fact of the world to change." "We all have our karma," an old man told me, echoing many others, as he sat in his house at the edge of town for our interview. "If we die young it's our karma; if we die old it's our karma. We have to be born, get old, hurt, and die. We're born and grow and hurt and die, and it's karma."

"I hear people in Europe and America don't believe in karma," another man listening in added. "But I don't believe that. I bet deep down they do. Karma is just so self-evident."[2]

No one professes disbelief in karma in Mae Jaeng. The reason people don't see *not* believing in karma as an option is that to them it is not a belief; it is a construct that organizes the world and has the kinds of self-evident qualities one might associate with common sense, the natural order, or universal truths. Karma is seen to explain everything. It is used to explain large and small events in Mae Jaeng, from a productive day at work to the devastating effects of a region-wide tsunami.

I went to talk to the head monk in Mae Wak outside of Mae Jaeng, the same monk who months earlier had told me about losing his wallet on the back of a motorbike, to ask more about karma. After I'd paid my respects and we sat down in the shade, he told me that karma may seem to work in mysterious ways, but only because people are too ignorant to see it all in play. If we practice more, if we know more, he said, we can see all the causes and all the effects of things that happen.

---

2. The pervasiveness of karma is often also downplayed in anthropological and religious studies of Buddhism. Charles Keyes suggests that karma is seen to work as a causal mechanism only in times of death or when other explanations are not forthcoming: "It is only when a condition is clearly beyond the ability of anyone to do anything to rectify it—and such conditions are actually rarely accepted outside of death—that one interprets it as having been a consequence of previous karma. Karmic theory, insofar as it involves utilizing supposed previous actions to explain present conditions, is drawn upon only for ultimate explanations—for an explanation that can be used when no other explanation (scientific or magical) satisfies" (Keyes 1983, 267). People in Mae Jaeng for the most part concurred in naming karma as the causal source for everything, along with rather than in competition with other kinds of explanations. It can be thought of as part of the "webs of significance" that make up the cultural fabric of everyday life (Geertz, *The Interpretation of Cultures*, 1973b). Sir Edward Evans-Pritchard made a similar point about the pervasiveness of cultural constructs in his discussion of witchcraft among the Sudanese Azande: "The web is not an external structure in which he is enclosed. It is the texture of his thought and he cannot think that his thought is wrong" (Evans-Pritchard 1976, 109).

A friend who had just come back from a meditation retreat at Wat Rampoeng in Chiang Mai told me what was considered an extension of the monk's sentiment: "If you meditate for a really long time you can even start to see your past lives!"[3]

Karma is used to explain present fortune (both good and bad) and is the religious reason for making merit. Periodically I would ask Mae Daeng what I could do around the house to help her out, which seemed important, since I wasn't paying an official monthly rent to stay there. Inevitably, each time I asked she told me that one thing I could do was to donate money to the wat on her behalf. I would hesitate and tell her that while I agreed it was a nice practice, I would rather give the money to *her* to spend on household goods. But to Mae Daeng, donating to the wat was a more worthwhile thing to do: "If you *tham bun*," she told me, "if you make merit well, you'll be born in a better life. A good life, with good status and more money. It's good for you, and good for me." I watched the way that Goy's friend who was staying with us presented money or gifts to Mae Daeng periodically, kneeling down on the floor in front of Mae Daeng and *wai-*ing her as she did, handing her an envelop with some bills in it or a box with a watch or similar contribution, and I would try to mimic her. I gave Mae Daeng money here and there in packets when I could, and she and I would go to the wat together to donate some of it.

Mae Daeng brought up the effects of her merit making in other ways, too: "I made merit well in my last life, so now I'm here," she told me. "And I've had the chance to meet you, that's from my merit."

While Sen continued to drink, and I and others continued to try to help him, I learned about karma and how it was understood to work in Mae

---

3. The reference to past lives and rebirth are tied to a local Thai cosmology that conceives of five fairly separate realms of sentient existence: at the lowest realm are the hells, where the negative effects of actions are expressed in a variety of macabre ways; the next highest realm is that of animals, who are thought to be ignorant; the next higher realm is that of ghosts (in Thai, *phi*), who are thought to wander around living out their leftover karmic attachments; the next realm is that of humans, who are thought to be lucky enough to be able to understand the Buddha's teaching but still suffer from corporeality; the highest realm is that of the heavens, where "angels" (*thewada*) live in various noncorporeal planes of pleasure. Existence in each realm can last thousands of years, but like all existence is inevitably impermanent, because of the effect of karma. Nirvana (*nibbana*) represents the extinguishing of all karma and is seen as outside these five realms of suffering. For more on Thai Buddhist cosmology see Buddhadasa 1990.

Jaeng. In interviews I heard hundreds of narratives about explanations for events, and in all these stories the role of karma was mentioned. It was brought up in the very first interview I had done with P'Dao, when she talked about the karma of Mae Daeng's husband, who had died at the family fire a few years earlier: it was his karma that he died, and she said it was the karma of Mae Daeng to be now living alone. Others talked about karma to explain deaths and accidents, including the Andaman tsunami, which had happened in recent memory, and even in the far North, I was told, had caused tables to shake and objects to fall off shelves. It was used to explain personal loss and good fortune alike.

Why did I win from the lottery ticket I bought at the temple? It's my good karma.

Why did he get into the accident? It was because he was drunk, and because of karma.

Why did the tsunami happen? If we think of science, then it was an earthquake, and if we think of Buddhism, it was the karma of those there.[4]

"It helps Mae Mon's karma," Pan told me in the back of a pickup truck a few months after Mae Mon had passed away, as we were heading home from a monastery celebration called *ngan poy*, held one hundred days after the death. I had asked him the meaning of the ritual: "It helps her get to heaven," he told me. Even after death, the effects of merit can be felt.[5]

---

4. Karma is usually not the only explanation for events, but it is almost always understood to be part of an explanation. There was a tendency in interviews to explain events through both proximate physical causes and distal, often karmic causes. Evans-Pritchard's (1976) observation that the Azande know well the physical aspects of cause and effect but also seek further explanations for why a particular event happened to a particular person is similar: the two kinds of explanations are seen as complementary rather than conflicting.

5. As with life, death is also explained through karma. When people use up the lot of karma that generated their present life, they die, and their overall karma propels them to their place of rebirth in one of the five Buddhist realms of existence: the realms of the hells, animals, hungry ghosts, humans, or heavens. Explaining death as having used up one's karma was a familiar refrain in interviews when I asked people to tell me why someone they knew had died. After the person being interviewed related an instance when a neighbor got sick and passed away, or a relative

Canceling Out Karma

Gaew was on her motorbike one night on the way home from the market when a drunk man driving a pickup truck ran into her bike. When Aung and I rushed to the hospital, we found her with only a scratch and a slight concussion; later she said lightly, "Well, that's my karma." When a friend of a friend in Bangkok had a car accident, karma was similarly brought up: "It's good," the friend said. "My friend can't walk right now, but now she's used up some karma, so she won't have it [negative karma] anymore in the next life."

One of the positive aspects of even bad things that happen to people is that a little bit of karma is thought to be used up. It is thought that getting new good karma is good, but the ultimate goal in Buddhist thought is to have no karma at all. It is only through having no karma that one is able to achieve nirvana. It is thought to be good to get rid of one's old karma: it doesn't always feel good, but it helps in the long run. People in Mae Jaeng are familiar with a popular *sutta* passage in which the Buddha at the time of his enlightenment relates karma as the force that constructs the experience of perpetual rebirths. He gains nirvana, the Buddhist goal, by finishing up his karmic stock. In the passage, the Buddha refers to his continued corporeal existence as a metaphorical house, and karma as its builder: "I have had numerous births. In vain have I sought the builder of the house.

---

got into an accident and died, I would ask, "Why do you think that happened?" and was told *"Mot kam*: her karma for this life ran out." Saying that one dies when one's karma is used up seems to suggest that the person had no more karma. In textual accounts in the Tripitaka, the extinguishing of karma is discussed not in terms of rebirth but in terms of enlightenment; but for most people in Mae Jaeng it refers less to overall karma being extinguished and more about the finishing of karma that propelled one to be born in his or her present life. When people die, then, they may have run out of that lifetime's worth of karma, and are thought to be reborn with the leftover karma generated from this and other lives. When most people think of being reborn they think of being reborn in the human realm, hopefully with more comforts than in this one, but no one knows. "I'll go to a good place," I heard most often when I asked what would happen after death, but I heard other thoughts, too. One old woman told me about a neighbor who bothered his family so much she was sure he would be reborn as a ghost and continue to torment them. Because all intentional action must bear its consequence, even if the karma that propelled one into the present life is used up, causing the individual to pass away, if the overall karma attached to the person is not completely extinguished, another being is born to bear it out. The accounting of karma as having run out at death but still left over to propel rebirth may seem to be a contradiction, but it is only an apparent one. It works as a way to explain the events of life and death.

Oh, the torment of perpetual rebirth! But I have seen you at last, O builder of the house. You no longer build the house. The rafters are broken; the old walls are down. The ancient mountain crumbles; the mind attains to nirvana. Birth is no more, for desire is no more."[6]

In this famous passage it is clear that getting rid of karma is a central religious goal. At the same time that one aspires to get rid of one's overall karmic load, however, the merit making that is so popular in Mae Jaeng is about creating karma, specifically good karma. Making merit is understood to propel positive karma, both in this life and the next. As I heard often when I asked about the reasons for merit, "I make merit so in my next life I'll be rich and powerful!" While karma and merit (*bun*) are conceptually the same, people rarely mention karma and merit in the same conversation. Merit is discussed as the positive creation of good future karma, while karma when discussed explicitly, usually is done so in terms of the present expression of demeritorious actions from past lives. The idea of creating good karma clearly suggests good effects: "Do good and meet with good," as the saying goes.

Following the religious ideal of not wanting to have any karma while at the same time actively seeking out good new karma draws attention to an analytical puzzle about Buddhist religious practice: if it's good to get rid of one's karma, why make new karma as merit? Merit increases positive experiences in the form of good karma, but it is thought that karma propels the cycle of suffering. The Buddhist goals of extinguishing overall karma and creating new good karma through merit making are both shared social ideals in Mae Jaeng, but they can appear contradictory, because every time merit is made, karma is made too. There is a conceptual gap: the more karma that one makes, even if it is "good" karma, the higher status one is thought to attain in the future, both in this life and in future births, both in the human and in the heavenly realm; but there is no way to attain so much "good" karma that one "ascends" to *nippan*, to nirvana. Gaining good karma does not lead one increasingly closer to and finally to reach nirvana. It is in part this theoretical impasse that inspired some Buddhist studies scholars to suggest that there are two "kinds" of Buddhism,

---

6. Hérold (1922) 1997. For more on nirvana in Buddhism see Steven Collins's *Nirvana and Other Buddhist Felicities: Utopias of the Pali Imaginaire* (1998).

with one oriented toward seeking out new karma and the other working to extinguish it.

Except for the truly enlightened, it is thought that no one knows the exact workings of karma, but people around me guessed all the time, and connected present actions to good effects in the future. The process of karma is complicated, and for most people it's practically unknowable, but it is not considered esoteric. The causal link between karmic action and karmic reaction is considered obvious. Its effects are felt in personal experiences, its positive accumulation is gained through omnipresent acts of merit, and the two are not often raised in casual conversation together. It was only when I started asking about the relationship between old karma and new merit that I heard people talk about their thoughts on the topic and realized how many different perspectives there are on the issue. I heard different answers from different people, but none pointed to exclusive, distinct soteriological paths.[7] Instead there was a sense of ambiguity, along with a confidence that getting rid of one's karma is good; also that making merit, regardless, is a worthwhile thing to do.

Reconciling the ideal practices of gaining positive karma in merit while also seeking a state of no karma took two general forms: (1) new good karma can be seen as canceling out (or minimizing) the accumulation of past bad karma, and (2) good new karma can be seen as practice in making no karma at all through emotional practice.

First, new good karma may cancel out bad old karma. Perspectives on this differ from person to person in Mae Jaeng, and even with the same person at different times.

"Can making positive karma now [*tham bun*] cancel out negative karma from earlier?" I asked a monk visiting our neighborhood monastery of Wat Ko from his monastery in Bangkok.

---

7. It is theoretically possible that a goal of not having any karma and a goal of making positive karma reflect different kinds of goals: Melford Spiro suggested as much when he said that most people follow what he called a "kammatic" path of Buddhism based on gathering good karma, while far fewer follow the difficult and exalted "nibbanic" path based on not creating any karma at all (1982). But most people in Mae Jaeng do not see it this way at all; even given the apparent contradiction, most people think of the positive karma gained through meritmaking as very much helping one on the long path to nirvana.

"No," he said. "There's no overlap in creating good karma and the effect of past bad karma. The bad karma must be expressed, now or in the future, regardless of what good you do now." He used a metaphor of salt in water to illustrate: "Let's say we think of salt as positive karma you just made, and water as your overall karmic load. Sometimes a little salt you just made is put into a glass that has just a little water, in the case of someone who has just a little past bad karma, and the salt changes the overall chemical makeup of the glass. And other times the same amount of salt, of good karma, is put into a glass overflowing with water, and the salt doesn't make much of a difference."[8]

I went to talk to Goy at her shop to ask her the same question. As usual I found her in the back of the store listening to a monk chant on the radio and reading a book about the *dhamma*. Goy, who read the most Buddhist texts of anyone I knew in Mae Jaeng, told me about a complex relationship between good and bad, past and present karma. At first she said the same thing the monk had told me: "No, it doesn't work like that. All your bad karma from the past must get worked out. And so you wait, through ten, twenty lives, doing good and waiting for your old past bad karma to use itself up, and then you are in *nibbana*, nirvana."

Later that night, though, when we were talking about it back at the house, Goy reconsidered: "Well ... actually it depends. The good new karma has to meet with the old karma, and they *khui gan*—they talk. If the old karma accepts the new karma, then it can change, for some people. But if it can't accept it then it can't, I think."

At this point Goy knew me well enough to refrain from just telling me to go talk to the monks about these difficult questions, and she knew I was interested in her take on the issue, but it wasn't something that she had already figured out a perspective on.

Unlike the confidence that people spoke with when they discussed issues of nonattachment and impermanence, the attitudes that people shared on the subject of karma were usually spoken without strong conviction. Karma is clearly real to people in Mae Jaeng, but its workings are not always clearly evident for ordinary (nonenlightened) people. One man

---

8. Although there are many textual articulations of karma, this monk's answer could be considered a formal, textually backed one; the same metaphor of salt and water he used, for example, can be found in the Anguttaranikya sutra.

I interviewed held his hands out to each side like a balance scale to illustrate the situation of making good new karma and extinguishing old bad karma. He said, "When you do good, say ten units of good karma"—he lowered one hand a bit to mimic the weight of merit—"then you have ten units less, say, of old bad karma." He raised the other hand the same amount. It was an interesting response, and I must have looked intrigued at the idea, because when he looked up and saw the curious expression on my face he said, "Oh, is that wrong?"

"Oh, I don't know!" I answered, "I'm just trying to learn about it."

He went on then, reconsidering: "Well, OK, it doesn't decrease your old past bad karma, but still, it can help. . . . Let's say you get into an accident and you're in a coma at the hospital. If you've made merit recently [good karma], you'd still be in the coma, but then you'd wake up, whereas if you hadn't made that merit [and therefore felt the fuller expression of the older bad karma], then you'd die."

Here karma is seen to mix less as a balance and more as a give-and-take that is differently expressed in experience. Analogies came up a lot when people talked about karma: metaphors of a feedback loop, of dilution in water, of balance beams, of personified karmic conversations and more were common. People constructed their own personal ways of thinking about karma.

What to me was the most interesting conversation about the possibility of old karma and new karma canceling each other out took place with Mae Daeng one night while one of her sisters, Mae Lah, and Mae Lah's daughter Niw were at our house cooking pork and vegetables on the fire. Niw was visiting from America for a few weeks, and I asked the three of them about the interaction of past and future karma.

Niw began: "Well, some people believe if you make good karma your old bad karma decreases, and some don't. It's fifty-fifty."

Her mother Mae Lah jumped in: "Actually, if you make merit your old bad karma is less, that's the true thing—"

Niw interrupted her, laughing: "See, she's one who believes the first!"

Mae Daeng agreed with her sister: "It's true, what Mae Lah says. I do good, I make merit, and I think I'll have less bad karma because of it."

Niw continued, "Hmmm, well, I don't believe like that—I don't think the overall karma is less when you do good."

Mae Lah said, explaining the difference in views, "Well, Mae Daeng and I were raised in the same family, so we think the same like that. My daughter here has been living away from home, off in Bangkok and out of the country, so she's developed her own ideas."

This conversation demonstrated to me how open the issue is for contestation; there are varying perspectives, and there is no automatic deference to some "authoritative source." Mae Daeng and Mae Lah both believed that making good new karma in the form of merit decreases, or cancels out, one's overall karmic load, and they aligned themselves with what they saw as the correct interpretation.

Karmic Emotion

A second way to approach the issue is to think of merit making as emotional practice in acting without karmic accrual. Classical Buddhist texts divide karma into three categories: (1) bright karma with bright ripening, (2) dark karma with dark ripening, and (3) neither dark nor bright karma, with neither dark nor bright ripening, that leads to the exhaustion of karma.[9] For the most part this works out clearly in practice: Good actions (that is, intentional actions, actions done with a particularly "good" affective intentionality) produce the first type of good karma: actions done with good intention produce good results. Bad actions (that is, actions done with a particularly "bad" affective intentionality) produce bad karma: actions done with bad intention produce bad results. The third category is trickier: actions done without intentionality do not create karma. Heightened, agitated emotions create karma, both good and bad, and acting without intentions does not. Intentional actions done with calm, non-desiring, nonattached feelings, however, while they still make some karma, are more connected to this third kind of action that produces no karma than are intentional actions done with feelings of desire and attachment. The Buddha is thought to have pointed to this connection between desire and karma at the end of his house-builder analogy: "I have had numerous births. . . . The ancient mountain crumbles; the mind attains to nirvana; birth is no more, for desire is no more."

---

9. From the *Majjhima Nikaya* 57, the Dog-Duty Ascetic (*Kukkuravatika Sutta*). Some sources also state a fourth kind: darkandbright karma with darkandbright ripening

The "builder" of the house is one's own karma, which in effect is one's own desires; the desire is part of the intention, or the emotion, behind action.[10] With intention come feeling states, and it is here especially that emotion comes into play. The "seed" of action that bears the karmic "fruit," I was told, in the common metaphor of a plant, is intent driven by desire, and desire (as hinted at earlier) is based on attachments and a longing for permanence. Acting with good intention produces good results, and acting with bad intention produces bad results. Acting without intention, on the other hand, means acting without desire. As I was told again and again, making merit is about acting with a certain emotional countenance, a particular affective demeanor. Bad karma is made with bad feelings at play, feelings that include selfishness, ill will, and robust emotion.

On the national Thai Buddhist holiday of Makhabucha, Gaew was in Chiang Mai and decided to go to the wat with some offerings. However, as she told me later, "I didn't make it to the wat because there were too many people. It's OK, I came home and *wai*-ed at home with good intention." It is the intention that creates the merit. I was reminded of the man who had told me that just throwing some food into a monk's bowl would not make merit; it had to be done with the right intention.[11] People did not toss money in the bin at the wat, for example; the bodily and emotional demeanor is always one of calmness. This connection between affect and effect is true for other areas of social life, too: food will taste good or not taste good, I was told, depending on the cook's mood when preparing the food. The efficacy of an offering at the wat is positively correlated with how selflessly it was made.

---

10. This emphasis on intention is the distinguishing feature of the Buddhist theory of karma. It differentiates Buddhist ideas about karma from the wider Hindu and Jain world in which Buddhism developed, where karma was thought to be accumulated through actions that (for Jainism) took on material form (Laidlaw 1995).

11. In Pali sources especially, but in Buddhism more generally, and especially compared with other karmic religions like Hinduism or Jainism, intention and with it emotional orientations are implicated in karma. Agency in Pali Buddhist traditions is more personal than the compassion toward all sentient beings found in the Mahayana traditions. Comparing the Mahayana Divyāvadāna with Pali texts, Rotman tells us that "unlike the Pali materials, the Divyāvadāna portrays the arising of this mental state as having less to do with the personal natures and predispositions of individuals than with the impersonal functioning and effects of conditioned existence" (2003, 564). Compared to "this notion of individuals being moved by an agency outside themselves," Pali Buddhist accounts conceptualize personal agency squarely within the individual, even as the "individual" is itself understood as an impermanent and insubstantial thing.

During a trip out to the mountains one weekend with Goy and some of her friends from her radio station, I was admonished for my enthusiasm about the beauty of the area. I commented profusely on how wonderful the area was, and the gratitude I felt to be there. "Be careful," Goy told me; "you don't want to feel too happy." When I asked her to explain, she told me, "Well, it's like sometimes when I make merit without expectation; at these times my mind feels happiness, it's very joyful. It's like a big bubble, and it gets bigger and bigger. But actually if you feel like that too much, it's not good."

A monk in Mae Jaeng elaborated on this sentiment: "Try to get out of the circle, try to stop your desire, your needs, your wants, stop your craving. Because these things will make you want to make [bad] karma." The craving and desire that go into attachment create actions that make karma, and the way to end karma is to act without craving, desire, and attachment.

A formal Pali Buddhist word related to emotion and volition is *cetanā*. *Cetanā* is best translated as desire or will, connecting intentionality with affect. Wants, desires, and feelings about events are the key components that produce karmic effects. An old, bedridden man I encountered, who was hard of hearing, illustrated this point when he told me that extinguishing desire is the most important Buddhist goal, "but," he went on, laughing, "even though I'm old and I can't hear much anymore, I still have desires, I still want sex, food, to have fun—maybe when I'm older it'll be easier to follow the path!"

Acting without desire is central to the Buddhist project. Calmness, acceptance, and letting go are all inscribed within practices that both gain merit and train one to act without strong intentions or desires, which is thought to be the kind of action that does not gain new karma at all. The monk in Mae Jaeng went on: "There are three ways to make good karma. One is to give: to people, the monastery, etc. The second is to follow the precepts: to not lie, steal, etc. The third is to sit in meditation, to control your mind. You work on your mind to be peaceful and calm."

A Knife, an Ambulance, and a Trip to the Hospital

Sen's illness came to a head a year and a half after his family first noticed he had a problem. I had finished my official fieldwork and returned to Chicago, but during summer vacation I booked a flight back to see my host family and friends. I had been in touch with Sen and Gaew during the months away from Mae Jaeng, and Gaew had kept me up to date on her brother's condition.

"We took him to the psychiatric hospital for a day," she told me at one point about six months after I'd left, "and he's stopped drinking, so he'll be OK." But then, a month later, she called again: "Never mind, now he's started again."

"His phone isn't working anymore," Aung told me when I landed back in Chiang Mai and gave her a call. "He stopped charging the battery. I tried, but I haven't talked to him in weeks."

When I got into Mae Jaeng I went to see Gaew. She was sitting in the front room of the shop, her younger brother was at school, her husband was at work, her parents were away in Chiang Mai on another Buddhist retreat, and her older brother Sen was sitting in his room. While I had been away her family had decided to stop selling liquor in the store; where the liquor shelf had been behind the desk there was now a large portrait of Khruba Si Wichai, a famous and charismatic Northern Thai monk from Lamphoon.

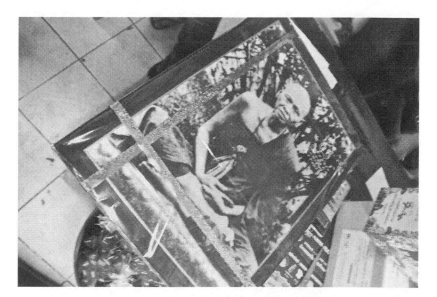

Figure 9. The image of Khruba Si Wichai, a famous charismatic Northern Thai monk, just before it was placed up on the shelf in Gaew's shop where whiskey used to be sold.

A handwritten note was taped under the portrait: "No Alcohol Sold Here." Gaew told me they put the picture of the monk up to remind customers who had wanted to buy liquor of the Buddhist precept against intoxication, with the hope that that would lessen their wish to buy it. We talked for a few minutes, and I asked about Sen. Instead of answering, she just looked up at me in silence and motioned for me to go out to his room at the back of the house.

I had never been in Sen's room and was nervous to go there now. The space was dark and silent when I entered. Sen was sitting in an old rocking chair in a corner with a blanket over him, almost a ghost. He had lost more weight than I thought was possible for a person to do, his arm bones visible and his cheeks sunken into his skull. He looked over at me with empty, hollow eyes. I tried to be cheerful, but I could feel myself starting to cry. I didn't know what to say.

"I'm fine, Julia," he whispered, and then, laughing weakly, "but my feet are swollen." From his feet up to his knees the tissue of his legs was enormous and purple. His stomach was bloated too, probably from a protein deficiency. I touched his leg. My fingers left a thick blotchy imprint after I had let go.

"No one comes in here at all anymore." Sen stared blankly into space. After a while there was a knock at the window. A hand reached up, holding a pack of cigarettes and two clear plastic bags of rice whiskey.

Sen didn't say anything as he took them from his little brother, but when I asked Gaew later, she told me, "Noi does that every day for him. Sometimes we put plates of food out by the door for him, too, but he usually doesn't eat them, and he doesn't talk to anyone."

"We want to bring him to the hospital," she continued. "Six months ago I got him to the psychiatric hospital in Chiang Mai, like that time I told you about, where they treat people with addictions, but he wouldn't stay. The doctor said he could come back to see him anytime—I want to take him there again, but he won't go." She finished with, "If he doesn't want to go, we can't make him. He's *duu*—so stubborn."

That night I stayed with Sen in his room, and he muttered incoherently in a half sleep the whole night. The next morning, Gaew, Pan, and I talked about what to do. Pan felt we couldn't do anything to help until Sen was willing to get help and accept the situation, using, as I was used to, the terms *tham jai* and *yom rap* when he talked about what Sen should do—to make the heart and "pick up" the responsibility to take care of himself. Pan continued, "At least we should wait until Mae San and Paw Nui get back to Mae Jaeng from Chiang Mai in a week. *Jai yen.*"

"I think we need to do something now," I said. "He'll never admit he needs help, and if we don't do anything he'll die." Gaew was torn between Pan and me: she agreed with me that something needed to be done but knew how difficult, if not impossible, it would be to do it. We left the decision up to her, and she decided to try to get him medical attention. That night, she and I went to the house of Sen's childhood friend Ban to see if he would help force Sen into an ambulance. Gaew may have used the energy I brought with me from my arrival to motivate herself, and I went with her ambivalently. I had a nagging feeling that, as an anthropologist, I shouldn't be interfering in the lives of my "subjects." But my concern for my friend's health outweighed my professional concern for maintaining what I thought of as an appropriate distance from his personal life. The image of Sen's hollow eyes and puffy yellow skin were already starting to haunt me. I was still thinking at this point of my interviews as the "real" research, and my friendship with Gaew and Sen only relevant in the downtime of my own personal life. I didn't realize then that their lives were more telling about the emotions of making the heart in Mae Jaeng and living Buddhism than the interviews I had so carefully and thoroughly collected.

Ban was checking his Facebook while watching over his family's shop when we arrived. Gaew and I sat down and told him about Sen's condition. He agreed to help, and we went to gather two more friends as well. Our plan was to accost Sen early the following morning, force him into a hospital ambulance that Chai would arrange to have waiting in front of the house, and take him to the psychiatric doctor in Chiang Mai.

But Sen seemed to have foreseen what was about to happen from the way that Gaew and I were putting some things in a bag in his room in preparation for the trip. At seven o'clock the next morning the five of us approached his bedroom. Sen had locked the door. After a few tries Ban succeeded in knocking it down. Sen was sitting up in his bed holding a large sharp kitchen knife in his hands, looking at us as though possessed.

"I'm . . . NOT . . . going to the hospital," Sen said slowly, holding the knife out at us. Everyone immediately backed away, scared, looking at him warily, now from the corner of the room. It wasn't clear that he had the strength to use the knife, but in his apparent state, we thought he might be capable of anything. We tried to talk to him, but he just glared at us and repeated his adamant refusal.

Finally, "I don't want to mess with a knife," Ban said. The others agreed. Within minutes, they slowly filed out. We had failed.

"Let's wait until Mae San and Paw Nui come home," Pan suggested again over breakfast, after Sen had fallen back asleep in a daze. Paw Nui and Mae San were away at one of their regular *yo reh* retreats in Chiang Mai.

"*Jai yen yen*," Pan said: "let's be cool-hearted, patient, and give him some time. If he doesn't want to be in the hospital, we can't make him."

It seemed like an impossible situation. Everything I had learned so far about emotion and action in Mae Jaeng suggested that being calm, cool, and accepting of events with a patient demeanor was the correct attitude to have. It seemed to work for every other situation in Mae Jaeng, but in this case it didn't seem to be working.

"We've got to do something, and now," I told Gaew, and she agreed.

"We could go to the police and have them do it . . . but people in town will see," she continued. "It's not fair to him, to have others watch him being taken away. Maybe we should wait until night. Or not."

Gaew and I went to the police station at the center of town and had a talk with the police chief, who like everyone else knew the family.

"Sen needs to go to the hospital," she told him, describing the problem in a short, matter-of-fact way. "He needs to, but he won't go. We need your help."

"Really? Oh, wow . . . OK." The police chief seemed surprised and a little discombobulated. Like most people in Mae Jaeng, he knew Sen; they were the same age and had spent time together during Sen's childhood summer vacations at home.

"But, I don't know what we can do if someone's holding a knife to us," the police chief said when Gaew finished explaining the situation. "See if you can get the knife away from him, and we'll put him into an ambulance."

I went back to Sen's room. He was half sleeping. I lay down next to him and pretended to sleep too.

"It's nice in here," he mumbled. "I don't want to go anywhere." I could see the knife lying just above his head on the headboard of the bed, his arm outstretched toward it. After he was asleep I slowly reached over and took the knife, put it in my back pocket, climbed over him, and left the room. I showed it to Gaew, my hands shaking. We went back to the police chief and told him we were ready.

I was still shaken from the incident and didn't think I could stand going back into the room to watch the police, so I waited out in the front of the shop with Noi while five uniformed policemen stormed through to the back of the house. Gaew told me later that the scene was awful to witness, that she felt so bad for her brother as he desperately looked for the knife and, realizing it wasn't there, became scared of the people in the room. When the officers came out of the house they carried Sen, unmoving, on a stretcher with them. He was gazing blankly at the sky, the straps of the mat holding him down.

In the ambulance the air was optimistic; Sen was finally getting to the hospital for medical attention. We had won, the alcohol had lost, and Sen would be OK again. Gaew directed the driver to the Rongpayaban Suan Prung, Chiang Mai's psychiatric and addiction hospital that Sen had visited a half a year earlier, and where the head doctor had said Sen could come anytime. But it was Saturday, and the head doctor wasn't there. And when the attending staff at the entrance looked at Sen, they told the ambulance driver to move on: "His eyes are too yellow. He's too far gone. Take him to a regular hospital."

"They just want to avoid any more work this weekend," Sen's cousin muttered under his breath in the back of the ambulance, but we drove out of the psychiatric hospital grounds to Nakhon Ping, one of the two public hospitals serving the Chiang Mai region. There, the staff were happy to admit him, and we were soon waiting for a doctor. Sen was put into a large room with about two hundred other patients, all within a few inches of each other and in various states of duress. He was a little awake but mostly unconscious, lying on his bed without speaking.

"It'll be about three days until the alcohol leaves his system," the intake doctor said, "and he should be fine." His parents showed up about three hours after he had arrived: they had wanted to finish their Buddhist exercises at the meditation center they had been staying at in Chiang Mai, so as to make merit for him before seeing him. I was angry with them for taking so long to arrive, because, to me, making merit and finishing their chants couldn't be as useful as being there in person for their son. But they thought differently, and I think that Gaew did too. The air was celebratory that afternoon; even though he didn't like it, Sen was finally going to get the help he so desperately needed.

But Sen's prognosis slowly got worse. Blood tests were taken that showed a whole range of problems. His potassium levels were down, and they weren't rising with the supplemental injection.

"He has cirrhosis of the liver. It's irreversible," the doctor said matter-of-factly. "See this bloating here?" pointing to Sen's legs. "That's what this is. His liver is failing. And he has hepatitis A and B."

"He could live a year or two or three," the doctor said the next day, when all the tests were in, "or he could die in just a few months. It's hard to say." Sen slowly regained consciousness and started talking haltingly, but he could barely walk. Family and friends stayed with him in shifts, one of the requirements the hospital had for patients staying in the private room to which his parents had had him moved. Mentally he still appeared blurry, but he seemed somewhat better, even managing to smoke a cigarette that his father had sneaked in for him against the hospital's no smoking policy.

When he was coherent enough to talk a few days later I asked if he missed alcohol, and he said he didn't. "I miss my brother," he said, "Tell Noi to come visit."

"Noi doesn't want to visit," Gaew said when I told her about the conversation that night. "Sen doesn't actually want to see Noi. He wants Noi to come because Noi usually brings him his whiskey and cigarettes. Noi's scared of not doing what he says."

When it became clear that Sen wouldn't be receiving any more cigarettes or alcohol, his mood worsened. He refused to eat, and the hospital staff pumped him with salt water. Gaew visited the wat at the edge of the hospital grounds each morning, where she made merit on Sen's behalf, handing out donation envelopes with Sen's name on them for us to sign and transfer merit to him. Days went by, and Sen didn't eat and the doctor didn't visit; in the busy public hospital the doctor would come by only once a week instead of daily. Sen was getting weaker and weaker. Even the nurses were getting worried, and their talk turned to the weeks Sen had left rather than months or years. After a week deteriorating in the hospital Sen was moved to Chiang Mai's expensive, private hospital, Chiang Mai Ram. He was barely coherent, occasionally mumbling unintelligibly and looking around with a seemingly distraught, resigned, semi-incredulous look.

At Chiang Mai Ram, Sen began falling in and out of consciousness, spending more and more time asleep or incoherent. Hospital staff put a feeding tube up his nose and attached multiple machines to him to monitor his vital signs. At this point, Sen started hallucinating: he elaborately and silently consumed a piece of imaginary cake and would look up and touch his forefinger to his thumb repeatedly. Gaew pieced together that the latter gesture was Sen ashing an imaginary cigarette. The prognosis got worse. "Already 98 percent, almost 100 percent of his liver has failed," the doctor said. "Sometimes cases like this can get better, but not this one." Gaew, Noi, Aung, their parents, and a few other relatives and friends began crowding into the hospital room. Some stayed at the house where I was staying in Chiang Mai or another friend's house for the night, while others camped out in the hospital waiting room.

Over the following week, while we waited, Gaew and her family alternated between a pragmatic calmness and a vacant, distressing calmness. Sen's mom cried for a few short, quiet moments.

"It's my karma that this happened," she said to me as we were sitting at the hospital watching Sen sleep. "It's my karma that I had a son that this happened to. It's his karma that it happened to him. And it's your karma too, Julia, that you met someone like this." Sen's dad stared into space a lot. It was apparently news to everyone that their son, their brother, their friend would not be getting better. "I figured he would drink and then eventually one day stop, either on his own or with help, and then he'd be fine," Sen's mother told me.

Gaew and her family seemed calmer than I would have imagined they would be. The calmness was real and deep, permeating the emotional environment at the hospital and at home. It wasn't because other people were watching; it wasn't about suppressing an emotion. It was about trying to feel OK about a situation, no matter how awful.

Only Mae Daeng's niece Dee, visiting from England, told me, "They didn't do anything at all for him. Why didn't they make him stop drinking earlier? If my kid got into trouble like this I would do anything. I would yell at them. I would scream at them. But they didn't do anything." She was so upset, and I didn't know what to say. I had been living in Thailand for a while now and wasn't used to Dee's emotional demeanor. She paused and said, "But it's the way of people around here." Everyone other than Dee, including Gaew, Paw Nui, Mae San, Noi, Pan, their cousins, and Sen's friends, didn't talk much about the situation or try to think too much about it; they were there, and they cared, but they felt that it was better, both for themselves and for Sen, to not feel too upset. When I tried to talk to them about it they told me not to—not only to not talk about it, but to not think about it; to just be.

After Sen had been in the new hospital for a week—he was now surrounded by a mess of tubes and barely awake at all—a nurse pulled his parents aside. She said the same kind of thing that others had told them, about him not getting better, but was more firm about it, and less open to the chance of a different outcome. "You know," she stated with a weak, concerned smile, "the doctors won't tell you this, because it's their attitude to keep working on someone with everything they've got, and they want to make more money. But I've seen this kind of thing before, and I'm sorry. You could keep him here for weeks, for months even, but he's not going to make it. I've seen it. Livers don't get better. You have to *tham jai*. Bring him home, let him be comfortable."

After this frank conversation, Sen's parents decided to bring him back to Mae Jaeng.[12] They couldn't afford the hundreds of thousands of dollars required for a liver transplant at a top hospital in Bangkok, and even if they could, the waiting list would likely be too lengthy. And given the direness of Sen's condition, he wouldn't be considered a good candidate because he was already too far gone.

"He'll be more comfortable at home," Sen's mom said to us, echoing what the nurse had told her. The next morning Sen and the rest of us left. Sen managed to wake up long enough to joke weakly with the ambulance staff on the way back to Mae Jaeng, not really sure what was going on. On the road back over the mountains I saw Chai's car heading in the direction of Chiang Mai—he'd stayed away until then, unsure how much to get involved, but when Gaew called to tell him we were returning, he turned his car around and followed us back.

---

12. Moving patients back to their home at the end of life is a common practice in Thailand. Scott Stonington discusses it in *The Spirit Ambulance: Life, Death, and Ethical Tension in Thailand* (in press), along with the issues it raises for integrating cultural diversity in health care practices with increasing biomedical advances that can often artificially extend life.

When we arrived at the Mae Jaeng hospital, his friends crowded around his stretcher. Chai, Aung, Ban, and all the others, about ten or fifteen people in total, talked to him quietly, joking around. He was still hallucinating a bit from his alcohol withdrawal, and in between fits of semiconscious sleep he smiled, in half recognition of the people surrounding him. He was installed in a private room in the hospital, where his family and friends could visit easily.

The day after the return to Mae Jaeng was Sen's birthday. Everyone gathered around and sang to him, even though he was completely unconscious and his hands were tied down to the side of the bed to keep him from reflexively flinging off the tubes in his body. It was Noi's birthday too, the brothers having been born on the same day of the year. Sen's father, Aung, Gaew, and I took Noi out to dinner, in an attempt to cheer him up. Noi was twelve years old. We ate cake and sang "Happy Birthday."

"Noi, I want you to know, you can be whatever you want to be when you grow up," his father told him in a serious tone as we were eating the cake. "You can be a doctor, an artist . . . anything you want to do, you can do." I had never heard Paw Nui talk like that before, or since. He seemed to want to remind Noi that he didn't have to end up like Sen. Noi just nodded. We all went back to the hospital after dinner.

Sen stayed at the local hospital for another week. His friends stopped by his bed regularly. Chai helped to lift him when he had to change beds or move rooms. The local spirit doctor Nan Jon was brought in from his office at the back of the hospital to see Sen. I had met him earlier and had interviewed him then; it was the same doctor who had told Mae Daeng to float the small boat when she was sick.

Nan Jon came into the room where Sen lay semiconscious, and Chai raised Sen's body so that Nan Jon could place thick leaves around him. Paw Nui, Mae San, Gaew, Noi, Chai, Aung, Sen's nurse friends, and I all stood crowding the edges of the small room. Nan Jon held a wick with water at the ends and chanted in a low Pali cadence as he flicked the wick at Sen. He circled Sen, singing, and after about twenty minutes he was done. He left the hospital room, and Sen's parents were alone with him again. "What just happened?" I asked. "What did Nan Jon do?" The doctor was getting the spirits of the alcohol to detach from Sen's own life spirits, Paw Nui told me, using the Tai *khwan* to refer to the force that is part

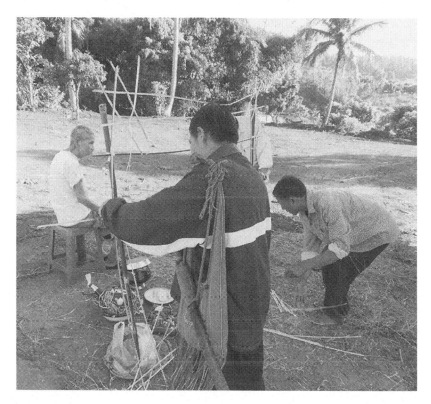

Figure 10. A spirit doctor in Mae Jaeng behind the town hospital, preparing to help a patient.
Photo by Padungpon Sukontamontrikul.

of what is thought to make up a living person.[13] "They're gone now." The act of detaching had begun.

After Sen was brought back to Mae Jaeng his friends seemed quiet, trying to laugh and take it lightly. Everyone else did the same. While he was at the hospital, Sen's friend Ban said softly, "We have to *ploy* [let go]." His

---

13. *Khwan* is a regional concept referring to the souls of the self and can be thought of as a kind of personified "wit," which can be lost (as in "one has lost his wits" or "one has lost her *khwan*"). Rituals to call back the *khwan* are held regularly in this region. White strings are tied around wrists of those sick or about to travel to help keep their *khwan* together, as well as tied around the necks of newborn babies, motorcycle handles, car rearview mirrors, and even whole monastery buildings and village neighborhoods, for similar reasons. For more on *khwan* see Robbins, Cassaniti, and Luhrmann 2011. The designation "Tai" refers to an ethnic and language group of peoples in Northern Thailand, Laos, Burma, and southern China.

friends agreed. All the things I had learned about and witnessed in Mae Jaeng about letting go, staying calm, and making the heart seemed to fold in together. It was karma that created the situation, and making the heart meant coming to terms with that. "We have to accept what has happened," I heard again and again. "We have to *tham jai*."

I talked to Moh Bom about whether Sen could get better: "*Anicca* . . . ," he told me, "do you know that word? It means impermanence. Everything changes. Nothing is permanent."

But his statement wasn't a defeatist one: it was a way to think about helping him. "Sen will do better here," I overheard Paw Nui saying to Gaew and Noi later. "The hospitals didn't do anything. Now that he's back in Mae Jaeng, we can make more merit for him." Everyone I knew seemed to be making merit for Sen once his health issues were known around town. His father was at the wat every morning; Mae Daeng stopped by to let them know she had just come from doing the same. Even Jerapong, the pastor at the church in Ban Ko Tao, brought a group to pray over Sen's bed. The emotional tone the week following Sen's return to Mae Jaeng was in many ways the same one I had gotten used to during my fieldwork: calmness, acceptance, and letting go, but it was heightened, more explicit, and more articulated in practice.

Those in Sen's immediate family mentioned his condition only rarely in those days back in town. Other than the first day on returning to Mae Jaeng, when they closed the shop for the day, they continued on with their lives and didn't seem to show many outward signs of stress. "Sen finished his karma," his cousin told me as we got on a motorbike to go home the evening of the second day back. "*Gert gae jep tai*," I heard again and again: "We're born, we grow, we hurt, and we die." "He had a certain amount of karma," Sen's mother said, "and it's gone now. We're born, we grow, we hurt, and we die." Mae Daeng said, "Everyone is born, grows old, and dies. I tell myself this." It is a common Buddhist phrase, and she said it to feel better, to tell me to feel better, and to calmly accept the situation. But it wasn't the acceptance of giving up; it was the acceptance of making the heart, and such actions were understood to help themselves, and also to help Sen.

For a year, I had struggled with what seemed like Gaew and her family's failure to do anything to help Sen, and with not knowing or asking what Sen's problems were. But slowly I came to realize that the practices of nonattachment, making the heart, and calmly letting go got results; the problem hadn't been that people around Sen were following them, but that they weren't following them enough. They had wanted Sen to be a certain way, and he had wanted to be a certain way, but it wasn't the way things were.

When Sen returned home from the hospital after another week there he was moved into the common room upstairs, outside his parents' bedroom door. They moved back from the house they had moved to after Mae Mon's death and started staying home more. Accepting the situation, whether Sen lived or died, was the crucial thing. Gaew had wanted him to be a certain person, a certain kind of brother, and she had fought with herself and him to make him so. She had wanted her life to be a certain way, and while she was successful at it, in most senses her brother had been causing her stress and created problems for her; and she let all this go when Sen came back from the hospital.

I was staying at the house, sleeping in Gaew's room, when Sen first returned home, as Pan was out of town for work. The first night her brother was back from the hospital, around midnight, Gaew and I had a long talk, and she shared her feelings with me.

"I *wish* I had forced him to go to the hospital earlier," she said. "Some night we were out when he was really drunk, like that time at Loy Krathong up the hill, I should have put him in the pickup truck and told him we were going home but driven to Chiang Mai instead." She was uncharacteristically distraught. But after a while she geared her emotions to the future.

"I've decided I'm going to close down the shop," she said. "I hear a 7–Eleven is coming to Mae Jaeng, and we could never compete with them. They blare lights all day and night, and the workers have to wear uniforms and stand up the whole time. . . . I've been meaning to close down the shop anyway. Business is bad—after we stopped selling alcohol in the store no one came in here anymore. I'm going to *ploy*, I'm going to *wang*, I'm going to let go of everything. I'm going to live a peaceful life."

Sen's health issues revealed the complex workings of karma, not just for himself but also for his family and friends. Karma was raised explicitly by his mother and others around him, when they said it was their karma to know someone going through something like this, and my karma too for the same reason. It was brought up implicitly in the ways that people made sense of Sen's problems; he was suffering in part because of the natural consequences of failing to let go of attachments. And it was especially inscribed within ideas about the right course of action to take, the one to get results: to accept, let go, and live a peaceful life.

Conclusion

Acting Apart

After the doctors released him from the hospital Sen spent a year lying in bed upstairs in the common room of his family home. After the first few weeks he became more coherent and conscious, and soon he was able to talk a bit again and take the medicine the doctors gave him. After a few months a masseuse friend started to come by three times a week to massage his legs, which had atrophied after the bloating had subsided. And after almost twelve months in bed Sen reached for a lamp and, finding himself too far away to turn it on, hoisted himself up and crawled over to it. Soon he was walking again, cooking food, and even riding a bicycle (in a wobbly circuit) on the street in front of the house. The doctor called his recovery a miracle, and others did too, but no one thought too hard about it, preferring to "let it go" and see what the future would bring.

Seven years after Uncle Anurak died in a motorcycle accident during my first summer in Mae Jaeng, and two years after Sen first began his downward plunge into alcoholism, Gaew closed down their family shop. She bought a food cart and on the street in front of the family home started selling noodles to passersby. The shop space was rented out to neighbors. A 7–Eleven had opened up down the block at the Mae Jaeng gas station, but Gaew's mother's sister owned the new store, so the money it made stayed in the family. It was one of the few 7–Elevens I had seen in Thailand that didn't sell alcohol. At first I thought that Gaew's decision to close the family shop had been a kind of caving in to encroaching businesses, or a fizzling out of personal ambition. But with the money being generated from the changes, she was even more successful in business than before; she was more comfortable financially as well as mentally.

After finishing my PhD, I had taken a few months off to go back and see my friends again in Mae Jaeng. The town seemed different; there were more cars, and more stores. Mae Daeng was getting older, and was thinking of retiring her market stall and taking care of her garden full time. Goy continued to run her stationery store, tutoring children and DJ-ing at the local radio station on the side when she had time. She seemed even more relaxed and content than before. Gaew's and Sen's friends didn't seem to come by their house as much, but they still stopped in from time to time. Life was continuing on as usual.

I was dealing with my own issues of trying to let go of my graduate student identity, find a job, and embrace another phase of life. "I'm not sure what to do next," I told Aung and Sen as the three of us sat down to bowls of noodles from Gaew's stand in front of their house. "The job market for academics is hard; there aren't a lot of good options out there." We talked comfortably and casually, as if time hadn't passed at all. "Tham jai," Aung said, and Sen nodded in agreement.

That night Sen and I talked about his year as an invalid and his recovery. I asked him what he remembered from his time at the hospitals, and he told me he didn't remember any of it. "I just remember when Chai was there and lifted me when some doctor came in, that's all I really remember," Sen said. "The rest is blurry." We talked a little bit about what had happened at the hospitals, and then started watching TV, a show about people in Bangkok doing stories on strange people living in the countryside. At one point he turned to me and said, "You know, it's our karma that we know each other. We must have known each other in our last life, that's why we've met now. Otherwise how would we meet, you living all the way in America and me out in this little town in Thailand."

I remembered what Gaew had told me about good things being more likely to happen to people whose hearts are able to let go, as an explanation of karma: "People with good, content hearts can *ploy*," she'd said, "they can let go, so they'll feel OK; they can change their life and adapt so their life will become good again."

I repeated to Sen what Gaew had said, and he nodded. "Yeah. Gaew's a good example of that, too. When the store wasn't doing well, she didn't stress, she *ploy*. She let it go. She closed the shop and opened the noodle stand. And she's good now."

"But what if you steal a lot of money?" I asked, intrigued by the idea that letting go creates positive effects not just internally but in the "real world," too. "What if you spend the rest of your life lounging on a beach somewhere living off what you took? You're feeling *sabai*, good and comfortable, right?"

"No," he corrected me. "If you've stolen money you don't feel comfortable in your heart. You might feel comfortable in your body, but your heart isn't well. You're stressed, worried about the bad karma you've made, that you're feeling, worried about the police. . . ."

Much later that night we talked more, as the rest of the town slept. Sen said, "Julia, do you know why I've gotten better?"

"Not really. Why?"

"Gaew thinks it's because of her, that she started doing things right. My dad thinks it's because of him, that he started making merit for me more. You think it's because you helped me. Even the pastor at that church from Ban Ko Tao, when he brought his friends to come to pray for me in the hospital, they think they got God to help me. All that helped. But I know the real reason. The real reason I got better is that I did it myself: I let go."

Through his own doing and that of those around him, Sen seemed to have come around to being able, finally, to let go. He didn't struggle with his feelings as he had before; he accepted them. When Chai came by the shop, they nodded hello to each other. When Pan passed by him in the house he didn't grimace. He sat comfortably with his parents and let them offer their Buddhist chants to him. His friends stopped by to visit, and although his troubles didn't end, they became easier for him.

Sen's illness and the ways his family and friends dealt with it help to make sense of a local psychological model of health and well-being. This model points to the letting go of attachments as part of a broader system of cause and effect. It helps explain why Sen got sick, and why he recovered. The interviews I did helped add support to the breadth of the model. The comparative work in the Karen Christian community suggested that attitudes and emotions in Mae Jaeng are not shared in the same way everywhere, but are instead constructed in and through social context. In the end, though, the interviews and comparative contrasts served as supplements to the much more personal and informal encounters with people whose lives I got to know in Mae Jaeng. It was through individuals and my observations and interactions with them over time that I learned the most about how people craft subjectivities in everyday life through engagements with local religious ideas. More broadly, the ways they live Buddhism suggest new theoretical perspectives for the study of culture, mind, and religious practice. These broader conclusions revolve around the central purpose of this work: it draws attention to a local model of personal agency.

Agency

Personal agency refers to the ability to create change and act in the world. Most Western, universalizing assumptions about agency view it as something akin to free will—the ability of an agent to act apart from the constraints of his or her culture. In the postmodern heyday of the 1990s, "agency" served as a focus of critical culture study, and was approached in terms of "resistance" and "rebellion," rendered in opposition to structure to act against what was seen as the hegemonic norms of one's culture (Ortner 1997). But a new way altogether of thinking about agency has begun to emerge more recently, one that attends to the ways it is formed *through* rather than *apart from* culture (Laidlaw 2014; Ortner 2006; Desjarlais 2001; Mahmood 2005; Menon 2002). Culture provides a kind of mental toolkit, in this sense, for action. The possibilities that culture offers are always implicated in the ways that people act; Lila Abu-Lughod's example of Bedouin women's poetry (1999) shows how people make use of available cultural forms to express feelings that can only be made sense of through the particular values and social structures of the place. Bourdieu calls this the habitus, the "structured, structuring dispositions" that we draw from in making the possible real (1990, 52). We're always constrained by our habitus, Bourdieu points out; we always choose our course of action through the options available to us, even as these options shift and grow over time (2011, 1977). If we think of culture as providing the conceptual space for possibilities, it makes sense that we can't act apart from culture any more than we can choose to breathe something other than the air around us. Richard Shweder has made a similarly strong claim when he says that culture and psyche "make each other up" (1991). Breaking down the artificial distinction of an internal "real self" existing apart from an external social reality is the goal of cultural psychology; following it means to see more clearly how personal agency works within social life.

The local model of personal agency that I have been drawing is different from models in the social sciences that privilege action on the world. It is oriented to particular kinds of emotional practices and religiously influenced ontological assumptions that work to create effects through the acceptance of change. The model looks like this: everything in the world changes (from the teaching of *anicca*, impermanence), and so getting stuck on some idea or person or thing will bring suffering because it won't last; being aware of this impermanence and detaching from these things thus brings about positive results, and this detaching is practiced through the cultivation of calm, cool, affective orientations (as captured by making the heart in *tham jai*). Merit making and the work of karma serve to mobilize the effects of these practices, and socially reinforce the idea that following them creates positive change.[1]

This model in one sense could be thought of as being about acceptance. But when one thinks of agency in the traditional sense of external action on the world, accepting things that happen could incorrectly be seen as

---

1. This agency is practiced especially in the making of merit. When I had asked Mae Daeng and Goy why they made merit, they both offered explanations that were about giving, and for both of them it seemed to be a good thing to do, but it also seemed that Mae Daeng's and Goy's responses reflected two different interpretations: one spoke of wanting things, like health for oneself and one's children, and the other spoke of a feeling of practicing calmness and nonattachment. I sometimes heard people in Chiang Mai almost derisively say that most Thai people don't make merit for the "right" reasons: "they just want things—good grades, money—they don't understand the meaning," and it seemed that Mae Daeng's explanation fit this "incorrect" form and that it was more common than Goy's reason. For a while, the apparent discontinuity bothered me: when people made merit did they just "want" things in return? From what I had read about Buddhism, that wasn't its essence. Did people make merit to gain or to let go? Neighbors and family members commented to me that Goy and Mae Daeng were opposites in character, one chatty and cheery and the other quiet and somber, and their different attitudes about merit reflected their different personalities. But though different in personality and justifications for merit making, they went to the monastery together and at least behaviorally made merit in the same manner. I came to

reflecting a kind of passivity, or a lack of control.[2] In a conversation I had with an American colleague about impermanence in Mae Jaeng this very conclusion was suggested to me: "Maybe by being aware of change," she had said, "it means that people know they don't have control in their lives." The image of the poor rural farmer, disenfranchised by the political power machine of Bangkok or the global neoliberal economy, might serve to reinforce this impression. But the opposite, in effect, is the case, and appreciating alternative models of personal agency helps to explain why this is so. The more one is able to let go of affective attachments, the more one becomes in control of his or her life and surroundings. Acting apart doesn't just mean acting against culture but also and in important ways acting through it.

This picture of agency has theoretical implications for the way we think about the interaction of culture and the mind more broadly. Most of the findings in the psychological sciences about the ways the mind works are based on studies done in American or European contexts (or even just on educated, well-off university students who serve as the subject pool for psychological research), but we are now beginning to understand that to make sense of the human mind we need to take psychological diversity seriously.[3] Such an awareness means that we need to correct universalizing (Western-based) assumptions about the mind. Attention to the psychology of personal agency as inscribed within rather than without culture allows us to do this, and from it we can learn about a whole range of related psychological processes and practices. As the anthropologist Laura Ahearn says, it is important to study "how agency may differ from society to society, and how these conceptions might be related to notions of personhood and causality" (2001, 113).

---

understand that their two explanations were intertwined: part of gaining means letting go; it is practice in nonattachment; and nonattachment helps one to get what one wants.

2. E.g., Spiro 1982; see Almond 1988 and Cassaniti 2006 for an overview of the historical emergence of this, and Anderson (1983) 2006, Kamala 1997, and Winichakul 1994 for an analysis of the role political interests in the region took in constructing ideas of Buddhist practice.

3. In the field of psychology, agency is often discussed most often in terms of personal control, drawing from Seligman's ideas of learned helplessness (1975; Rodin, Schooler, and Schaie 1990). As with agency, personal control is usually understood to operate universally the same way for all people everywhere. Cross-cultural psychological research, however, has drawn attention to what has been called "secondary control" (emphasizing internal adjustment rather than the action on the world suggested by what is called "primary control") and has found this second kind of control to be relatively more common in Asian cultural contexts (Rothbaum, Weisz, and Snyder 1982;

Religion in Culture, Culture in Religion

In relating how people live Buddhist ideas in Mae Jaeng I have in a sense collapsed religion with culture; I have tried not to claim one idea to be "religious" and another "cultural." I have done this because although there are distinctions to be found in Mae Jaeng between the formal rituals of Buddhist practice and everyday "secular" activities like buying goods at the market or playing sports by the riverside, the distinction quickly fades when we draw back and approach the practicalities of everyday life and attend to religious ideas informing assumptions about the world that underlie human action.

The field of Buddhist studies has gone through a series of changes in its recent history. Buddhism is for the most part considered to be a religion, but at one point it was called something more akin to a philosophy (Rhys Davids [1896] 2007). The drive to see Buddhism as more of a philosophy than a religion is still found in the field of Buddhist studies, especially in popular books like *Confession of a Buddhist Atheist* (Batchelor 2011) or *The Bodhisattva's Brain: Buddhism Naturalized* (Flanagan 2013) that paint it as a scientific and rational human project. A host of historical and political purposes have propelled this attitude (I discussed some of them in the introductory chapter), but the field of Buddhist studies (and the field of religious studies more broadly) has recently moved in the direction of examining religious practices as they are lived "on the ground," in the context of lived experience (as in McDaniel 2011, Samuels 2010). Works in this more recent, "grounded" tradition examine how people interpret Buddhist

---

Shapiro 1987; Rosenberg 1990; Heckhausen and Schulz 1995). For studies that make use of this construction in a Thai setting see McCarty 1999 and Weisz et al. 1996, 1984. Most of this kind of work is done in the field of cross-cultural psychology and compares mental life in different cultural communities. Drawing large-scale distinctions about mental life in different regions of the world may be problematic, as they can lack the detailed cultural context that anthropological fieldwork offers, but in so far as it suggests a move away from universalizing assumptions toward a recognition and respect for psychological as much as cultural diversity, the purpose of this kind of cross-cultural psychological research is positive. Like anthropologists who approach agency within culture, such cross-cultural psychologists draw attention to psychological diversity. For psychological approaches that do make use of the term "agency" see Gruber et al. 2015. In the field of religious studies Pascal Boyer (2001) has suggested that his (Western) model of agency may be tied to Christian ideas of the divine and a personified God; this in turn suggests that different religious conceptions may inform different models of agency.

ideas in ways that quite often look different from what a more abstracted doctrinal reading of religious ideals might suggest. *Living Buddhism* adds to this trajectory by attending to lived practices and the ways that people make sense of ideas in their idiosyncratic personal and cultural ways. But it also represents a divergence from this trajectory, incorporating what are often considered to be "doctrinal" Buddhist ideas squarely into the meaning systems that people work with as part of, rather than less relevant for, their everyday lives. By showing how people are living Buddhism in ways that are always personal and idiosyncratic but that also do make use of shared Buddhist ideas and ideals, I am in effect suggesting a move away from the study of authority or authenticity as residing in religious virtuosos and a move toward regular people as sources of knowledge about religious traditions.[4] Decentering the established authoritative voices of Buddhism allows us to see religious ideas as they are engaged in in a wider variety of settings and to a broader range of purposes than might be the case through other more traditional modes of religious interpretation.

I remember the Thai man in the coffee shop in Chiang Mai telling me that people in a "traditional" place like Mae Jaeng "know," but that at the same time they "don't know" about Buddhism. The man was pointing to a kind of tacky and nostalgic image of traditional life, conjuring the image almost of the "noble savages" living peacefully in their wise ignorance. The theoretical field of anthropology has thankfully now fairly fully broken down this illusion, and it is picking up the pieces to put together a much more diverse and honest picture of what people are like, and how they live. The man in the coffee shop was wrong about Mae Jaeng precisely because

---

4. This move is especially significant for the study of Buddhism, but it can also be made for other work on religious practice. I am not in a position to make broad claims about agency in Christianity based on my comparative case of Christian practice in the Karen community, but from conversations with people in the village it seems that agency may work quite differently there (Cassaniti 2012). Webb Keane addresses a dual process of agency in a Christian missionary context on the Indonesian island of Sambu; he writes that, contrasted to local non-Christian conceptions of agency, according to the missionaries' perspective, "in addition to the human interior, there is another locus of agency, namely God" (Keane 1997, 685). In his research on belief in Zambia, Thomas Kirsch makes a similar argument, pointing to the ways that, for the Christian Zambians he worked with, "belief was quintessential to their religious practices just because it had a certain performative power . . . namely the power to invoke spirits and, therefore, to invest rituals with effectiveness" (Kirsch 2004, 701). For more psychological anthropological perspectives on Christianity in practice see Csordas 2011, 1990, Robbins 2007, and Luhrmann 2012, 2004.

people do know about Buddhism, but in a way that is both deeply historical and deeply contemporary, and are, like all of us, putting together the
pieces of religious and cultural ideas by making sense of them in the shared
practices of their everyday lives.

Why We Should Care

Paying attention to the ways that people live Buddhism is important
because it can teach us about the role that religion has in orienting conceptions about the way the world is set up and our place in that world, and
about how these conceptions in turn inform our own local models of cultural psychology and psychological functioning. While it may seem that
the planet is becoming less culturally diverse as global flows of ideas contribute to the eradication of languages, customs, and ways of living, at the
same time the diversity that does exist in the world is becoming more and
more apparent, often for the same reasons: the increasing ease of actual
and virtual travel and the exposure to difference that comes with it. The
picture of Buddhism in Mae Jaeng I have written about here is in many
ways a psychologically hegemonic one on a local level, but it is a counter-
hegemonic one at a global scale. It is hegemonic in that in Mae Jaeng there
is some room for diversity—as one person could choose the path of a spirit
medium or a monk, for example—but someone like Sen was not in a position to engage with a wide range of possibilities for succeeding in life in a
radically different way. Yet on a large, global scale, the model of agency I
have drawn is not at all hegemonic; to many people Buddhism represents
an alternative to the status quo, a way of doing things that is different from
what their own local established system might offer them.

Health workers and medical anthropologists are increasingly attending to some of the possibilities that Buddhist-inspired health care might
suggest, among them mindfulness-based therapies that draw from Buddhist theories about time and perception.[5] In Thailand, as is the case everywhere, the dominant biomedical establishment is driven by practices that
are considered to be scientific and global (or *etic*) rather than religious and

---

5. E.g., Williams and Kabat-Zinn 2011; Barry 2014; Cassaniti 2014a, 2014b. I address this issue
more fully in forthcoming work as it pertains to mindfulness practices in Southeast Asia.

local (or *emic*). As is the case for most ideas, however, the ones that are felt to be global are actually crafted in particular times and places and as such incorporate particular ideas about the person and the body, and are then transported elsewhere, where they may not have as much traction. Medical practices are no different; they are global, but global in particular ways that are usually Western, rich, and urban. The doctors in the city hospitals that Sen visited were virtually all Buddhist, and in their informal if not formal assessments were influenced by the same Northern Thai Buddhist ideas about health that Sen and his family were. And yet, for the most part Sen's doctors and the dozens of other regional doctors I've spoken with since then favor health treatments that are particularly "not Buddhist," inscribed in a social world of professional hierarchy. Patients and their families are typically reluctant to speak up about preferred treatment strategies. It is only if and when local ideas about health and well-being are rearticulated as "modern" and "scientific" that they have a chance of entering into actual formal health practice. I hope this changes, and there are signs that it might actually be changing; but as it stands today, religion and medicine still occupy largely separate spheres of specialization. Doctors need to know how to communicate and interact with the personal cosmologies and histories of patients in order to meet their needs, but too often doctors through their training lack this particular kind of localized cultural capital. Modern medicinal health workers should not try to compete with local healing techniques informed by religious perspectives but (like most of the patients they see) embrace them, developing techniques aimed at understanding and helping individual patterns of psychological functioning. A separation between biomedical technologies and local religious cosmologies may in fact be unnecessary, if not unwarranted, as evidence mounts that a more explicit inclusion of local ideas about what it means to be well can help more people live happier and healthier lives (Jenkins, forthcoming; Jenkins and Barrett 2004; Belzen 2004). The goal of such interventions should not be to extract them from culture into a supposedly acultural repertoire of science, but rather to incorporate meanings within variable cultural constructs into a larger repertoire of possible methodologies.

Taking psychological diversity seriously in the end serves most centrally to broaden the realm of the possible. Part of the reason that the model of personal agency I have drawn attention to works is that it functions within a larger system of Buddhist thought and social reinforcement in Thailand. In attending to the cultural context of lived Buddhism in one community, I am not saying that Buddhism works only in Thailand; but I am also not making a "theological" argument that Buddhism stands to work universally as the general "cure for what ails us." What I want to say is that understanding the psychological underpinnings of Buddhism in practice in one place helps us to open up the realm of what is possible in our own lives. It widens our habitus, adding to the cultural toolkit at our disposal and increasing the range of possible ways of living; and it allows us to see a certain type of deep psychological difference that we otherwise might not see if we generalize psychology across time and space. The cultural psychology that underpins the Buddhism I have drawn attention to here isn't that of Buddhism everywhere; it is particular to time and place and to the people who make use of ideas they associate with the religion as they live their lives. And this always is and has been the case. This connection between abstract shared religious ideas and concrete physical bodies is thus central to what I have suggested here.

The purpose of an ethnography is to illuminate enough about a different way of living in the world that readers may question their own assumptions about how they live; I have tried to do this for a new way to think about the interaction of culture and the mind by drawing attention to the cultural psychology of Buddhist practice in Thailand. The construction of mental lives lived through the engagement with culturally meaningful ideas has in this sense been the larger theoretical goal of my project.

One way to think of this book is as "Living Buddhism" where living is an adjective, a qualification for the type of Buddhism discussed in the text. It is my hope that for the reader it now appears more as a verb instead, as practices that people engage in culturally as they make Buddhist teachings part of their lives. The experience of everyday life in Mae Jaeng is not a somehow imperfect reflection of a real or true Buddhism of abstract thought; it is uniquely grounded in experience just as every other personal experience is, and combines the material of our biological selves with shared ideas and ideals. The psychology of the human being is always one that is inscribed within, and through, experiences that can only be partially and imperfectly abstracted. An objective fact is always also a subjective one; Buddhism in practice shows how this is so in Thailand.

GLOSSARY

The following terms are transliterated from the Thai, unless otherwise noted as Pali, *kam muang* (Northern Thai), or Karen.

anatta. (Pali) Buddhist term referring to the absence of a stable self; one of the three ti-lakkhana, or Three Characteristics.

anicca. (Pali) Buddhist term referring to impermanence, uncertainty, and change; one of the three ti-lakkhana, or Three Characteristics. Pronounced *anit chang* in Thai.

arom. Mood.

Asanha Bucha. Holiday celebrating the first sermon of the Buddha.

chedi. Stupa.

chuey. Dispassion, unroused equanimity.

dham- (*dhamma* in Pali). The Laws of Nature and the Buddhist teachings about the laws of nature.

dukkha. (Pali) Buddhist term referring to dissatisfaction or suffering.

farang. Westerners of European ancestry.

Guan Im. Goddess of compassion (Chinese *Avalokiteshvara*).

gurlah. (Karen) soul, glossed as the Thai *winyan*.

gert gae jep dai. To be born, grow, hurt, and die. A common phrase used to talk about karma.

jai. The heart-mind, used frequently in metaphoric idioms to describe affective states.

jai ron. Roused and impatient (lit.: "hot heart").

jai yen. Calm and relaxed (lit.: "cool heart").

jey (or **che**). A Chinese form of vegetarianism in which one refrains from eating not only meat but also garlic, onions, alcohol, and other stimulants.

jow mae. A guardian spirit.

kam (*kamma* in Pali, *karma* in Sanskrit). Karma; moral action and its consequences

kam muang. (Northern Thai) Northern Thai language or dialect (*kham muang* in Central Thai).

kathoey. A Transgender, transsexual, transvestite, or effeminate gay male.

khraw. Karma, luck, fortune, and fate, believed to meet one in the future, often negative.

khriat. Serious, stressed.

khwam ruu suuk. Feeling.

khwan. "Spirit," or vital force, a kind of personified "wits," a pan-Tai belief.

kreng jai. Deferential respect (lit.: "awe-struck heart").

loy. To float away.

Loy Krathong. Festival of lights, usually held in November, in which people float lanterns in the night sky.

mae. Mother. Also used to refer to older women, towns, rivers, and other place names in Northern Thailand.

mae chee. Female nun.

mai thiang. Instability, a colloquial Thai term to refer to *anicca*.

Makhabucha. Celebrating the first assemblage of followers of the Buddha.

muang. (Northern Thai) Referring to Northern Thai people (*kon muang*) (also means "city" in Northern Thai).

na. Flat rice fields common to Northern Thai farming, compared with *rai*, the sloped rice fields of the upland Karen.

nam jai. A helpful, kind heart (lit.: "water heart").

Nibbāna. (Pali) Nirvana; Buddhist enlightenment (*nipphan* in Thai, *nirvana* in Sanskrit)

Panyajan. The book of the Ecclesiastes in the Old Testament

phi. Ghost, spirit.

phra. A Buddhist Thai monk.

Phra Upakhut. *Muang* name for the spirit monk appeased during Loy Krathong.

plaek jai. Astonished (lit.: "strange heart").

plong. To lay down a burden.

ploy (or *ploy wang*). To let go, to not take something to heart.

sabai jai. A comfortable and satisfied heart.

sai sin. White thread (often on the wrist) used to call together the *khwan*.

samsāra . The continual cycle of life and death of earthly existence.

Sangha. (Pali) The Buddhist community ("Song" in Thai).

Songkran. The Thai New Year held every April.

tah guh law guh law. (Karen) Useless; to not have benefit.

tham bun. To do good, to make merit (*punya* in Pali).

tham dii dai dii, tham chua dai chua. "Do good meet with good, do bad meet with bad."

tham jai. To come to terms (lit.: to "make the heart").

thewada (also *thep*). A spirit, often translated as "angel" thought to reside in the heavens.

tok jai. To be surprised or scared (lit.: "the heart falls").

vinaya. Buddhist code of conduct or discipline, based on the Vinaya Pitaka.

wai. Thai greeting of respect, a slight bow with one's hands pressed together in front of their body; also to pay respect to the Buddha.

wan phra. "Monk day," "Buddha day," a weekly day of heightened religiosity.

wihan. Teaching hall (*vihan* or *vihara* in Pali and Sanskrit).

winyan. Spirit, or soul (*vinyan* in Pali).

yom (or *yom rap*). To accept, to come to terms with something; to receive or pick something up, figuratively and emotionally.

yo rey. A Japanese Buddhist sect practiced locally in Mae Jaeng that focuses on the power of the Buddha.

References

Abu-Lughod, Lila. 1999. *Veiled Sentiments: Honor and Poetry in a Bedouin Society*. Updated ed. Berkeley: University of California Press.

Ahearn, Laura M. 2001. "Language and Agency." *Annual Review of Anthropology* 30, no. 1: 109–37.

Almond, Philip C. 1988. *The British Discovery of Buddhism*. Cambridge: Cambridge University Press.

Anderson, Benedict. (1983) 2006. *Imagined Communities: Reflections on the Origin and Spread of Nationalism*. London: Verso.

Appadurai, Arjun. 1996. *Modernity at Large: Cultural Dimensions of Globalization*. Minneapolis: University of Minnesota Press.

Assanangkornchai, S., K. Conigrave, and J. Saunders. 2002. "Religious Beliefs and Practice, and Alcohol Use in Thai Men." *Alcohol & Alcoholism* 37, no. 2: 193–97.

Assanangkornchai, S., N. Sam-Angsri, S. Rerngpongpan, and A. Lertnakorn. 2010. "Patterns of Alcohol Consumption in the Thai Population: Results of the National Household Survey of 2007." *Alcohol & Alcoholism* 45, no. 3: 278–85.

Bamber, Scott. 1998. "Medicine, Food, and Poison in Traditional Thai Healing." *Osiris* 13, no. 1: 339–53.

Barry, B. 2014. *The Mindfulness Revolution*. Boston: Shambhala Publications.

Batchelor, Stephen. 2011. *Confession of a Buddhist Atheist*. New York: Spiegel & Grau.

Belzen, J. 2004. "Spirituality, Culture and Mental Health: Prospects and Risks for Contemporary Psychology of Religion." *Journal of Religion & Health* 43, no. 4: 291–316.

Benedict, Ruth. 2005. *Patterns of Culture*. Reprint, New York: First Mariner Books. First published 1934.

Bodhi, Bhikkhu, ed. 2003. *A Comprehensive Manual of Abhidhamma: The Abhidhammattha Sangaha of Ācariya Anuruddha*. Seattle: Buddhist Publication Society, Pariyatti Editions.

Boonmongkon, P., and Peter Jackson. 2012. *Thai Sex Talk: The Language of Sex and Sexuality in Thailand*. Chiang Mai, Thailand: Mekong Press.

Bourdieu, Pierre. 1977. *Outline of a Theory of Practice*. Cambridge: Cambridge University Press.

——. 1984. *Distinction: A Social Critique of the Judgement of Taste*. Cambridge, MA: Harvard University Press.

——. 1990. *The Logic of Practice*. Cambridge: Polity Press.

——. 2011. "The Forms of Capital." In *Cultural Theory: An Anthology*, edited by Madden I. Szeman and T. Kaposy, 81–93. Boston: Wiley-Blackwell.

Bowie, Katherine. 2008. "Standing in the Shadows: Of Matrilocality and the Role of Women in a Village Election in Northern Thailand." *American Ethnologist* 35, no. 1: 136–53.

——. 2011. "Polluted Identities: Ethnic Diversity and the Constitution of Northern Thai Beliefs on Gender." In *Southeast Asian Historiography: Unraveling the Myths; Essays in Honour of Barend Jan Terweil*, edited by Volker Grabowsky, 112–27. Bangkok: River Books Press.

Bowlby, John. (1969) 1983. *Attachment*. Vol. 1 of *Attachment and Loss*. 2nd ed., reprint. New York: Basic Books.

——. 1973. *Separation: Anxiety and Anger*. Vol. 2 of *Attachment and Loss*. London: Hogarth Press.

——. 1980. *Loss: Sadness and Depression*. Vol. 3 of *Attachment and Loss*. London: Hogarth Press.

Boyer, Pascal. 2001. *Religion Explained: The Human Instincts That Fashion Gods, Spirits and Ancestors*. New York: Basic Books.

Briggs, Jean L. 1970. *Never in Anger: Portrait of an Eskimo Family*. Cambridge, MA: Harvard University Press.

Buddhaghosa, Bhadantacariya. [430 CE] 2003. The Path of Purification: Visuddhimagga. Onalaska, WA: Pariyatti Publishing.

Buddhadasa, Bhikkhu. 1989. *Me and Mine: Selected Essays of Bhikkhu Buddhadasa*. Edited by Donald K. Swearer. Albany: SUNY Press.

——. 1990. *The Buddha's Doctrine of Anatta*. Bangkok: Vuddhidamma Fund.

——. 1992. *Paticcasamuppada: Practical Dependent Origination*. Nonthaburi, Thailand: Vuddhidamma Fund.

——. 2009. "Karma in Buddhism: A Message from Suan Mokkh." In *Rethinking Karma: The Dharma of Social Justice*, edited by Jonathan Watts, 3. Chiang Mai, Thailand: Silkworm Books.

Burnard, Philip, and Wassana Naiyapatana. 2004. "Culture and Communication in Thai Nursing: A Report of an Ethnographic Study." *International Journal of Nursing Studies* 41, no. 7: 755–65.

Butler, Judith. 1999. *Gender Trouble: Feminism and the Subversion of Identity*. Reprint. New York: Routledge. First published 1990.

Campos, J. J., R. G. Campos, and K. C. Barrett. 1989. "Emergent Themes in the Study of Emotional Development and Emotion Regulation." *Developmental Psychology* 25, no. 1: 394–402.

Carlisle, Steven. 2012. "Creative Sincerity: Thai Buddhist Karma Narratives and the Grounding of Truths." *Ethos: The Journal of Psychological Anthropology* 40, no. 3: 317–40.

Carstensen, L. L., D. Isaacowitz, and S. T. Charles. 1999. "Taking Time Seriously: A Theory of Socioemotional Selectivity." *American Psychologist* 54, no. 3: 165–81.

Cassaniti, Julia. 2006. "Toward a Cultural Psychology of Impermanence in Thailand." *Ethos: The Journal of Psychological Anthropology* 34, no. 1: 58–88.

——. 2012. "Questioning 'Belief': Agency and the Other in Christianity and Buddhism." *Ethos: The Journal of Psychological Anthropology* 40, no. 3: 297–316.

——. 2014a. "Buddhism and Positive Psychology." In *Positive Psychology of Religion across Cultures*, edited by Chu Kim-Prieto, 101–24. New York: Springer Press.

——. 2014b. "The Rural DJ." In *Figures of Southeast Asian Modernity*, edited by Joshua Barker, Erik Harms, and Johan Lindquist, 123–25. Honolulu: University of Hawai'i Press.

——. 2015a. "Asanha Bucha Day: Boring, Subversive, or Subversively Boring?" *Contemporary Buddhism* 16, no. 1 (May): 224–43.

——. 2015b. "Intersubjective Affect and Embodied Emotion: Feeling the Supernatural in Thailand." *The Anthropology of Consciousness*. Forthcoming.

Cassaniti, Julia, and T. M. Luhrmann. 2011. "Encountering the Supernatural: A Phenomenological Account of Mind." *Religion and Society* 2, no. 1: 37–53.

——. 2014. "The Cultural Kindling of Spiritual Experiences." *Current Anthropology* 55, no. 10: 333–43.

Chladek, Michael. Forthcoming. "Defining Manhood: Buddhist Monasticism as Ideal Masculinity in Thailand." *Rian Thai: International Journal of Thai Studies as part of ENITS*.

Chuchuhnjitsakun, Lisa. 2004. *Ruanglaojakphucow: Chiang Mai; Rongpim Fungfa* [Narratives from the hills]. Chiang Mai: Rungfa Press.

Cohler, B. J. 1982. "Personal Narrative and the Life Course." In *Life-Span Development and Behavior*, vol. 4, edited by P. Baltes and O. G. Brim, 205–41. New York: Academic Press.

Collins, Steven. 1982. *Selfless Persons: Imagery and Thought in Theravada Buddhism*. Cambridge: Cambridge University Press.

——. 1990. "On the Very Idea of the Pali Canon." *Journal of the Pali Text Society* 15:89–126.

——. 1998. *Nirvana and Other Buddhist Felicities: Utopias of the Pali Imaginaire*. New York: Cambridge University Press.

Condominas, Georges, and Gehan Wijeyewardene. 1990. *From Lawa to Mon, from Saa' to Thai: Historical and Anthropological Aspects of Southeast Asian Social Spaces*. Canberra: Department of Anthropology, Research School of Pacific Studies, Australian National University.

Cook, Joanna. 2010. *Meditation in Modern Buddhism: Renunciation and Change in Thai Monastic Life*. Cambridge: Cambridge University Press.

Csordas, Thomas J. 1990. "Embodiment as a Paradigm for Anthropology." *Ethos* 18, no. 1: 5–47.

———. 1994. *The Sacred Self: A Cultural Phenomenology of Charismatic Healing*. Berkeley: University of California Press.

———. 2011. "Embodiment: Agency, Sexual Difference, and Illness." In *Companion to the Anthropology of the Body/Embodiment*, edited by Frances E. Mascia-Lees, 137–56. Chichester, UK: Wiley Blackwell.

Davis, Richard. 1984. *Muang Metaphysics: A Study of Northern Thai Myth and Ritual*. Bangkok: Pandora.

De Silva, Padmasiri. (1979) 2000. *An Introduction to Buddhist Psychology*. Lanham, MD: Rowman & Littlefield.

Desjarlais, Robert. 2001. "Culture and Consciousness in South Asia." *Transcultural Psychiatry* 38, no. 4: 515–20.

Dicks, Andrew. 2006. "Homosexuality in Northern Thailand: Culture, Identity, and Community." Unpublished undergraduate thesis, University of Wisconsin–Madison.

Doniger O'Flaherty, Wendy, ed. 1980. *Karma and Rebirth in Classical Indian Traditions*. Berkeley: University of California Press.

Dumm, Thomas. 1999. *A Politics of the Ordinary*. New York: NYU Press.

Eberhardt, Nancy. 2006. *Imagining the Course of Life: Self-Transformation in a Shan Buddhist Community*. Honolulu: University of Hawai'i Press.

Ekman, Paul. 1994. "Strong Evidence for Universals in Facial Expressions: A Reply to Russell's Mistaken Critique." *Psychological Bulletin* 115, no. 2 (March): 268–87.

Ekman, P., W. V. Friesen, M. O'Sullivan, A. Chan, I. Diacoyanni-Tarlatzis, K. Heider, R. Krause, et al. 1987. "Universals and Cultural Differences in the Judgments of Facial Expressions of Emotion." *Journal of Personality and Social Psychology* 53, no. 4: 712–17.

Elinoff, Eli. 2014. "Sufficient Citizens: Moderation and the Politics of Sustainable Development in Thailand." *Political and Legal Anthropology Review* 37, no. 1: 89–108.

Engel, David M., and Jaruwan S. Engel. 2010. *Tort, Custom, and Karma: Globalization and Legal Consciousness in Thailand*. Stanford, CA: Stanford Law Books.

Evans-Pritchard, E. E. 1976. *Witchcraft, Oracles, and Magic among the Azande*. New York: Oxford University Press.

Flanagan, Owen. 2013. *The Bodhisattva's Brain: Buddhism Naturalized*. Cambridge, MA: MIT Press.

Formosa, Bernard. 1998. "Bad Death and Malevolent Spirits among the Thai Peoples." *Anthropos* 93: 3–17.

Foucault, Michel. 1980. *The History of Sexuality*. New York: Vintage Books.

Frijda, N. H. 1988. "The Laws of Emotion." *American Psychologist* 43, no. 5: 349–58.

Fuhrmann, Arnika. 2009. "Nang Nak Ghost Wife: Desire, Embodiment, and Buddhist Melancholia in a Contemporary Thai Ghost Film." *Discourse* 31, no. 3: 220–47.

Gay, Volney. 2003. "Passionate about Buddhism: Contesting Theories of Emotion." *Journal of the American Academy of Religion* 71, no. 3: 579–604.

Geertz, Clifford. 1960. *The Religion of Java.* Chicago: University of Chicago Press.

———. 1973a. "Deep Play: Notes on the Balinese Cockfight." In *The Interpretation of Cultures: Selected Essays*, 412–54. New York: Basic Books.

———. 1973b. *The Interpretation of Cultures: Selected Essays.* New York: Basic Books.

Gladwell, Malcolm. 2010. "Drinking Games." *New Yorker*, February. http://www.newyorker.com/magazine/2010/02/15/drinking games.

Goffman, Erving. 1959. *The Presentation of Self in Everyday Life.* New York: Doubleday/ Anchor.

Gray, Christine Elizabeth. 1986. "Thailand, the Soteriological State in the 1970's." PhD diss., University of Chicago.

Gregg, Melissa, and Gregory J. Seigworth. 2010. *The Affect Theory Reader.* Durham, NC: Duke University Press.

Gross, J. J. 1998. "The Emerging Field of Emotion Regulation: An Integrative Review." *Review of General Psychology* 2, no. 3: 271–99.

Gruber, Craig, Matthew Clark, Sven Hroar Klempe, and Jaan Valsiner. 2015. "Constraints of Agency." *Annals of Theoretical Psychology* 12.

Haberkorn, Tyrell. 2011. *Revolution Interrupted: Farmers, Students, Law, and Violence in Northern Thailand.* Madison: University of Wisconsin Press.

Haidt, Jonathan. 2006. *The Happiness Hypothesis: Finding Modern Truth in Ancient Wisdom.* New York: Basic Books.

Hall, Rebecca. 2008. "Of Merit and Ancestors: Buddhist Banners of Northern Thailand and Laos." PhD diss., University of California, Los Angeles.

———. Forthcoming. "Between the Living and the Dead: The Three-Tailed Funeral Banner of Northern Thailand." *Ars Orientalis.*

Hayami, Yoko. 2004. *Between Hills and Plains: Power and Practice in Socio-religious Dynamics among Karen.* Kyoto Area Studies on Asia, book 7. Melbourne: Trans Pacific Press.

Heckhausen, J., and R. Schulz. 1995. "A Life-Span Theory of Control." *Psychological Review* 102, no. 2: 284–304.

Hérold, A. Ferdinand. (1922) 1997. *The Life of Buddha.* Translated by Paul C. Blum.

Hickman, Jacob. 2007. "'Is It the Spirit or the Body?': Syncretism of Health Beliefs among Hmong Immigrants to Alaska." *Annals of Anthropological Practice* 27, no. 1: 176–95 (formerly *NAPA Bulletin*). Reprinted in *Sacred Realms: Readings in the Anthropology of Religion*, 2nd ed., edited by R. Warms, J. Garber, and R. J. McGee. New York: Oxford University Press, 2009.

Hirschkind, Charles. 2009. *The Ethical Soundscape: Cassette Sermons and Islamic Counterpublics.* New York: Columbia University Press.

Hochschild, Arlie Russell. 1979. "Emotion Work, Feeling Rules, and Social Structure." *American Journal of Sociology* 85, no. 3: 551–75.

Hovemyr, Anders P. 1989. *In Search of the Karen King: A Study in Karen Identity with Special Reference to 19th Century Karen Evangelism in Northern Thailand*. Uppsala, Sweden: Academiae Ubsaliensis.

Indrawooth, Prasook. 1999. "Dvaravati: A Critical Study Based on Archaeological Evidence. Bangkok: Silpakorn University.

Intasra, Wisin. 2006. *Trylak leh Priksmupbat. Samnakpim Thammada: Krungthep*. [The Three Characteristics]. Bangkok: Normal Press.

Jackson, Peter A. 1989. *Buddhism, Legitimization, and Conflict: The Political Functions of Urban Thai Buddhism*. Singapore: Institute of Southeast Asian Studies.

———. 2003. *Buddhadasa: Theravada Buddhism and Modernist Reform in Thailand*. Chiang Mai, Thailand: Silkworm Books.

Jenkins, Janis. Forthcoming. *Tangible Lives: Anthropological Studies of Culture, Mental Illness, and Extraordinary Experience*.

Jenkins, Janis, and Robert John Barrett, eds. 2004. *Schizophrenia, Culture, and Subjectivity: The Edge of Experience*. Cambridge Studies in Medical Anthropology. New York: Cambridge University Press.

Jessor, Richard, Anne Colby, and Richard A. Shweder. 1996. *Ethnography and Human Development: Context and Meaning in Social Inquiry*. Chicago: University of Chicago Press.

Ji, L., K. Peng, and R. Nisbett. 2000. "Culture, Control and Perception of Relations in Environment." *Journal of Personality and Social Psychology* 78, no. 5: 943–55.

Johnson, Andrew. 2014. *Ghosts and the New City*. Honolulu: University of Hawai'i Press.

Kamala, Tuyavanich. 1997. *Forest Recollections: Wandering Monks in Twentieth-Century Thailand*. Honolulu: University of Hawai'i Press.

Kãng, Dredge Byung'chu. 2012. "Kathoey 'in Trend': Emergent Genderscapes, National Anxieties and the Re-signification of Male-Bodied Effeminacy in Thailand." *Asian Studies Review* 36:475–94.

Keane, Webb. 1997. "From Fetishism to Sincerity: On Agency, the Speaking Subject, and Their Historicity in the Context of Religious Conversion." *Comparative Studies in Society and History* 30, no. 4: 674–93.

Keyes, Charles. (1977) 1995. *The Golden Peninsula: Culture and Adaptation in Mainland Southeast Asia*. Honolulu: University of Hawai'i Press.

———. 1983. "Merit-Transference in the Kammic Theory of Popular Theravāda Buddhism." In *Karma: An Anthropological Inquiry*, edited by Charles Keyes and E. Valentine Daniel, 261–86. Berkeley: University of California Press.

———. 1985. "The Interpretive Basis of Depression." In *Culture and Depression: Studies in the Anthropology and Cross-Cultural Psychiatry of Affect and Disorder*, edited by A. Kleinman and B. Good, 153–75. Berkeley: University of California Press.

———. 1989. "Buddhist Politics and Their Revolutionary Origins in Thailand." *International Political Science Review* 10, no. 2: 121–42.

Keyes, Charles, and E. Valentine Daniel, eds. 1983. *Karma: An Anthropological Inquiry*. Berkeley: University of California Press.

Kirsch, Thomas A. 1977. "Complexity in the Thai Religious System: An Interpretation." *Journal of Asian Studies* 36, no. 2: 241–66.

———. 2004. "Restaging the Will to Believe: Religious Pluralism, Antisyncretism, and the Problem of Belief." *American Anthropologist* 106, no. 4: 699–709.

Kitiarsa, Pattana. 2005. "Beyond Syncretism: Hybridization of Popular Religion in Contemporary Thailand." *Journal of Southeast Asian Studies* 36, no. 3: 461–87.

Knutson, Thomas J., Rosechongporn Komolsevin, Pat Chatiketu, and Val R. Smith. 2003. "A Cross-Cultural Comparison of Thai and US American Rhetorical Sensitivity: Implications for Intercultural Communication Effectiveness." *International Journal of Intercultural Relations* 27, no. 1: 63–78.

Kuan, Tse-fu. 2008. *Mindfulness in Early Buddhism: New Approaches through Psychology and Textual Analysis of Pali, Chinese, and Sanskrit Sources*. London: Routledge.

Laidlaw, James. 1995. *Riches and Renunciation: Religion, Economy, and Society among the Jains*. Oxford: Clarendon Press.

———. 2014: *The Subject of Virtue: An Anthropology of Ethics and Freedom*. Cambridge: Cambridge University Press.

Levy, Robert I. 1973. *Tahitians: Mind and Experience in the Society Islands*. Chicago: University of Chicago Press.

Loo Shwe, Thara (Saw). 1962. "The Karen People of Thailand and Christianity." Typescript, n.p., Rangoon.

Luhrmann, T. M. 2004. "Metakinesis: How God Becomes Intimate in Contemporary U.S. Christianity." *American Anthropologist* 106, no. 3: 518–28.

———. 2006. "Subjectivity." *Anthropological Theory* 6, no. 3: 345–61.

———. 2012. *When God Talks Back: Understanding the American Evangelical Relationship with God*. New York: Vintage Books.

Lutz, Catherine. 1988. *Unnatural Emotions: Everyday Sentiments on a Micronesian Atoll and Their Challenge to Western Theory*. Chicago: University of Chicago Press.

Lutz, C., and L. E. Abu-Lughod, eds. 1990. *Language and the Politics of Emotion*. Paris: Maison des sciences de l'homme and Cambridge University Press.

Lutz, C., and G. M. White. 1986. "The Anthropology of Emotions." *Annual Review of Anthropology* 15:405–36.

Mahmood, Saba. 2005. *Politics of Piety: The Islamic Revival and the Feminist Subject*. Princeton, NJ: Princeton University Press.

Malinowski, Bronislaw. 1922. *Argonauts of the Western Pacific: An Account of Noiive Enterprise and Adventure in the Archipelagoes of Melanesian New Guinea*. London: Routledge & Kegan Paul.

Markus, Hazel R., and Shinobu Kitayama. 1991. "Culture and the Self: Implications for Cognition, Emotion, and Motivation." *Psychological Review* 98, no. 2: 224–53.

Massumi, Brian. 1995. "The Autonomy of Affect." *Cultural Critique* 31:83–109.

Mauss, Marcel. 1934. "Les techniques du corps." *Journal de Psychologie*. Reprinted in *Sociologie et Anthropologie* 32, no. 1: 3–4.

McAdams, D. P., R. Josselson, and A. Lieblich, eds. 2006. "Making a Gay Identity: Life-Story and the Construction of a Coherent Self." In *Identity and Story: Crafting Self in Narrative*, 151–72. Washington, DC: American Psychological Association.

McCargo, Duncan. 2004. "Buddhism, Democracy and Identity In Thailand." *Democratization* 11, no. 4: 155–70.

McCarty, C., John R. Weisz, K. Wanitromanee, K. L. Eastman, S. Suwanlert, W. Chaiyasit, and E. Brotman Band. 1999. "Culture, Coping, and Context: Primary and Secondary Control among Thai and American Youth." *Journal of Child Psychology and Psychiatry* 40, no. 5: 809–18.

McDaniel, Justin. 2008. *Gathering Leaves and Lifting Words: Histories of Buddhist Monastic Education in Laos and Thailand*. Seattle: University of Washington Press.

———. 2011. *The Lovelorn Ghost and the Magical Monk: Practicing Buddhism in Modern Thailand*. New York: Columbia University Press.

Menon, Usha. 2002. "Making Śakti: Controlling (Natural) Impurity for Female (Cultural) Power." *Ethos* 30, nos. 1–2: 140–57.

Menon, Usha, and Richard A. Shweder. 1998. "Kali's Tongue: Cultural Psychology and the Power of Shame in Orissa, India." In *Welcome to Middle Age! (and Other Cultural Fictions)*, edited by Richard A. Shweder, 139–88. Chicago: University of Chicago Press.

Mesquita, Batja, and J. Leu. 2007. "The Cultural Psychology of Emotion." In *Handbook of Cultural Psychology*, edited by S. Kitayama and D. Cohen, 734–59. New York: Guilford Press.

Miller, J. G. 1984. "Culture and the Development of Everyday Social Explanation." *Journal of Personality and Social Psychology* 46, no. 5: 961–78.

Moore, Christopher. 2006. *Heart Talk*. Bangkok: Heaven Lake Press.

Morris, Rosalind. 2000. *In the Place of Origins: Modernity and Its Mediums in Northern Thailand*. Durham, NC: Duke University Press.

Muecke, Marjorie. 1979. "An Explication of 'Wind Illness' in Northern Thailand." *Culture, Medicine and Psychiatry* 3, no. 3: 267–300.

Nisbett, Richard. 2003. *The Geography of Thought: How Asians and Westerners Think Differently: And Why*. New York: Free Press.

Obeyesekere, Gananath. 1990. *The Work of Culture: Symbolic Transformation in Psychoanalysis and Anthropology*. Chicago: University of Chicago Press.

Ortner, Sherry B. 1984. "Theory in Anthropology since the Sixties." *Comparative Studies in Society and History* 26, no. 1: 126–66.

———. 1997. *Making Gender: The Politics and Erotics of Culture*. Boston: Beacon Press.

———. 2006. *Anthropology and Social Theory: Culture, Power, and the Acting Subject*. Durham, NC: Duke University Press.

Payutto, Phra Prayudh. 1992. *Dependent Origination: The Buddhist Law of Conditionality*. Translated by Bruce Evans. Bangkok: Buddhadhamma Foundation.

———. 1995. *Buddhadhamma: Natural Laws and Values for Life*. Albany: SUNY Press.

Penth, Hans. 2000. *A Brief History of Lan Na: Civilizations of North Thailand*. Chiang Mai, Thailand: Silkworm Books.

Platz, Roland. 2003. "Buddhism and Christianity in Competition? Religious and Ethnic Identity in Karen Communities of Northern Thailand." *Journal of Southeast Asian Studies* 34, no. 3: 473–90.

Posner, Jonathan, James A. Russell, and Bradley S. Peterson. 2005. "The Circumplex Model of Affect: An Integrative Approach to Affective Neuroscience, Cognitive

Development, and Psychopathology." *Development and Psychopathology* 17, no. 3: 715–34.

Puaksom, Davis. 2007. "Of Germs, Public Hygiene, and the Healthy Body: The Making of the Medicalizing State in Thailand." *Journal of Asian Studies* 66, no. 2: 311–44.

Quinn, Naomi, and Jeannette Mageo. 2013. *Attachment Reconsidered: Cultural Perspectives on a Western Theory*. Palgrave Macmillan.

Rahula, Walpola. 1974. *What the Buddha Taught*. New York: Grove Press.

Rajadhon, Anuman. 1986. *Popular Buddhism in Siam and Other Essays on Thai Studies*. Bangkok: Thai Inter-Religious Commission for Development.

Rhys Davids, T. W. (1896) 2007. *Buddhism: Its History and Literature*. New York: G. P. Putnam's Sons.

Robbins, Joel. 2007. "Continuity Thinking and the Problem of Christian Culture: Belief, Time, and the Anthropology of Christianity." *Current Anthropology* 48, no. 1: 5–38.

Robbins, J., J. Cassaniti, and T. M. Luhrmann. 2011. "The Constitution of Mind: What's in a Mind? Interiority and Boundedness." *Suomen Antropologi, the Finnish Anthropological Society* 36, no. 4: 15–20.

Rodin, Judith, Carmi Schooler, and K. Warner Schaie. 1990. *Self-Directedness: Cause and Effects throughout the Life Course*. Hillsdale, NJ: Lawrence Erlbaum Associates.

Rosaldo, R. I. 1984. "Grief and a Headhunter's Rage: On the Cultural Force of Emotions." In *Text, Play, and Story: The Construction and Reconstruction of Self and Society*, edited by S. Plattner and E. Bruner, 178–95. Long Grove, IL: Waveland Press.

Rosenberg, M. 1990. "Control of Environment and Control of Self." In *Self-Directedness: Cause and Effects throughout the Life Course*, edited by J. Rodin, C. Schooler, and K. Schaie, 147–54. Hillsdale, NJ: Lawrence Erlbaum Associates.

Rothbaum, Fred, John R. Weisz, and Samuel S. Snyder. 1982. "Changing the World and Changing the Self: A Two-Process Model of Perceived Control." *Journal of Personality and Social Psychology* 42, no. 1: 5–37.

Rotman, Andy. 2003. "The Erotics of Practice: Objects and Agency in Buddhist Avadāna Literature." *Journal of the American Academy of Religion* 71, no. 3: 555–78.

Rotter, J. 1966. "Generalized Expectancies for Internal versus External Control of Reinforcements." *Psychological Monographs* 80, no. 1: 1–28.

Russell, James A. 1980. "A Circumplex Model of Affect." *Journal of Personality and Social Psychology* 39, no. 6: 1161–78.

Russell, J. A., and L. F. Barrett. 1999. "Core Affect, Prototypical Emotional Episodes, and Other Things Called Emotion: Dissecting the Elephant." *Journal of Personality and Social Psychology* 76, no. 5: 805–19.

Sahdra, Baljinder Kaur, Phillip Shaver, and Kirk Warren Brown. 2010. "A Scale to Measure Nonattachment: A Buddhist Complement to Western Research on Attachment and Adaptive Functioning." *Journal of Personality Assessment* 92, no. 2: 116–27.

Samuels, Jeffrey. 2010. *Attracting the Heart: Social Relations and the Aesthetics of Emotion in Sri Lankan Monastic Culture*. Honolulu: University of Hawaiʻi Press.

Seligman, Martin E. P. 1975. *Helplessness: On Depression, Development, and Death*. San Francisco: W. H. Freeman.

Shapiro, D., Gary W. Evans, and J. Shapiro. 1987. "Human Control." *Science* 238, no. 4825: 260–61.

Shweder, Richard. 1990. "Cultural Psychology: What Is It?" In *Cultural Psychology: The Chicago Symposia on Culture and Human Development*, edited by J. W. Stigler, R. A. Shweder, and G. Herdt. New York: Cambridge University Press.

———. 1991. *Thinking through Cultures: Expeditions in Cultural Psychology*. Cambridge, MA: Harvard University Press.

———. 1994. "'You're Not Sick, You're Just in Love': Emotion as an Interpretive System." In The Nature of Emotions: Fundamental Questions, edited by Paul Ekman and Richard J. Davidson, 32–44. New York: Oxford University Press.

———. 2003a. "Toward a Deep Cultural Psychology of Shame." *Social Science* 70, no. 4: 1109–30.

Shweder, R., and E. Bourne. 1984. "Does the Concept of the Person Vary Cross-Culturally?" In *Culture Theory: Essays on Mind, Self, and Emotion*, edited by R. Shweder and R. LeVine, 158–99. New York: Cambridge University Press.

Shweder, Richard, Jonathan Haidt, Randall Horton, Craig Joseph, Michael Lewis, and Lisa Feldman Barrett. 2008. "The Cultural Psychology of the Emotions: Ancient and Renewed." In *The Handbook of Emotions*, 397–441. New York: Guilford Press.

Shweder, Richard, and Robert A. LeVine. 1984. *Culture Theory: Essays on Mind, Self and Emotion*. Cambridge: Cambridge University Press.

Sinnott, Megan. 2004. *Toms and Dees: Transgender Identity and Female Same-Sex Relationships in Thailand*. Honolulu: University of Hawai'i Press.

Skilling, Peter, Jason Carbine, Claudio Cicuzza, and Santi Pakdeekham, eds. 2012. *How Theravada Is Theravada? Exploring Buddhist Identities*. Chiang Mai, Thailand: Silkworm Books.

Spiro, Melford E. 1982. *Buddhism and Society: A Great Tradition and Its Burmese Vicissitudes*. 2nd, expanded ed. Berkeley: University of California Press.

Stigler, J. W., R. A. Shweder, and G. Herdt, eds. 1990. *Cultural Psychology: The Chicago Symposia on Culture and Human Development*. New York: Cambridge University Press.

Stonington, Scott. Forthcoming. *The Spirit Ambulence: Life, Death, and Ethical Tension in Thailand*. Ithaca, NY: Cornell University Press.

Strauss, Claudia, and Naomi Quinn. 1997. *A Cognitive Theory of Cultural Meaning*. Cambridge: Cambridge University Press.

Streckfuss, David. 2011. *Truth on Trial in Thailand: Defamation, Treason, and Lèse-Majesté*. London: Routledge.

Swearer, Donald K. 1988. "Buddhist Virtue, Voluntary Poverty, and Extensive Benevolence." *Journal of Religious Ethics* 26, no. 1: 71–103.

———. 2004. *Becoming the Buddha: The Ritual of Image Consecration in Thailand*. Princeton, NJ: Princeton University Press.

———. 2010. *The Buddhist World of Southeast Asia*. New York: SUNY Press.

Thamarangsi, T. 2013. "Addiction Research Centres and the Nurturing of Creativity: Center for Alcohol Studies (CAS)." *Addiction* 108, no. 7: 1201–6.

Thavorncharoensap, M., Yot Teerawattananon, Jomkwan Yothasamut, Chanida Lertpitakpong, Khannika Thitiboonsuwan, Prapag Neramitpitagkul, and Usa

Chaikledkaew. 2010. "The Economic Costs of Alcohol Consumption in Thailand, 2006." BMC Public Health 10:323.

Tsai, Jeanne L. 2007. "Ideal Affect: Cultural Causes and Behavioral Consequences." *Perspectives on Psychological Science* 2, no. 3: 242–59.

Tsai, Jeanne L., Brian Knutson, and Helene H. Fung. 2006. "Cultural Variation in Affect Valuation." *Journal of Personality and Social Psychology* 90, no. 2: 288–307.

Tsai, J. L., F. F. Miao, and E. Seppala. 2007. "Good Feelings in Christianity and Buddhism: Religious Differences in Ideal Affect." *Personality and Social Psychology Bulletin* 33, no. 3: 409–21.

Turner, Victor Witter. 1969. *The Ritual Process: Structure and Anti-structure*. Chicago: Aldine Publishing Co.

Veidlinger, Daniel. 2006. *Spreading the Dhamma: Writing, Orality, and Textual Transmission in Buddhist Northern Thailand*. Honolulu: University of Hawai'i Press.

Webster, David. 2005. *The Philosophy of Desire in the Buddhist Pali Canon*. London: Routledge Curzon.

Weiner, Eric. 2008. *The Geography of Bliss: One Grump's Search for the Happiest Places on Earth*. New York: Twelve Books.

Weisz, John R., Karen L. Eastman, and Carolyn A. McCarty. 1996. "Primary and Secondary Control in East Asia: Comments on Oerter et al. 1996." *Culture and Psychology* 2, no. 1: 63–76.

Weisz, John R., Fred M. Rothbaum, and Thomas C. Blackburn. 1984. "Swapping Recipes for Control." *American Psychologist* 39, no. 9: 974–75.

Whorf, Benjamin Lee. 1956. "The Relation of Habitual Thought and Behaviour to Language." In *Language, Thought, and Reality: Selected Writings of Benjamin Lee Whorf*, edited by John B. Carroll, 134–59. New York: Technology Press of MIT and Wiley.

Wierzbicka, Anna. 1999. *Emotions across Languages and Cultures: Diversity and Universals*. Cambridge: Cambridge University Press.

———. 2013. *Imprisoned in English: The Hazards of English as a Default Language*. New York: Oxford University Press.

Wijeyewardene, Gehan. 1984. *Place and Emotion in Northern Thai Ritual and Behavior*. Bangkok: Pandora.

———, ed. 1990. *Ethnic Groups across National Boundaries in Mainland Southeast Asia*. Singapore: Institute of Southeast Asian Studies.

Wikan, Unni. 1990. *Managing Turbulent Hearts: A Balinese Formula for Living*. Chicago: University of Chicago Press.

Williams, J. Mark G., and Jon Kabat-Zinn. 2011. "Mindfulness: Diverse Perspectives on Its Meaning, Origins, and Multiple Applications at the Intersection of Science and Dharma." *Contemporary Buddhism* 12, no. 1: 1–18.

Wilson, Ara. 2004. *The Intimate Economies of Bangkok: Tomboys, Tycoons, and Avon Ladies in the World City*. Berkeley: University of California Press.

Winichakul, Thongchai. 1994. *Siam Mapped: A History of the Geo-body of a Nation*. Honolulu: University of Hawai'i Press.

Index

Page numbers followed by letters *f* and *t* indicate figures and tables, respectively.

Made in the USA
San Bernardino, CA
21 August 2019